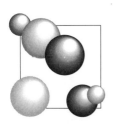

Molecular Aspects of Dermatology

Molecular Medical Science Series

Series Editors

Keith James, University of Edinburgh Medical School, UK
Alan Morris, University of Warwick, UK

Forthcoming Titles in the Series

Molecular Genetics of Human Inherited Disease *edited by* D.J. Shaw
Molecular Aspects of Bacterial Virulence *edited by* S. Patrick and M. Larkin
Molecular Techniques in Histopathology *edited by* J. Crocker

Other Titles in the Series

Plasma and Recombinant Blood Products in Medical Therapy *edited by* C.V. Prowse
Introduction to the Molecular Genetics of Cancer *edited by* R.G. Vile
The Molecular Biology of Immunosuppression *edited by* A.W. Thomson
Vaccine Design *by* F. Brown, G. Dougan, E.M. Hoey, S.J. Martin, B.K. Rima and A. Trudgett
Molecular and Antibody Probes in Diagnosis *edited by* M.R. Walker and R. Rapley

Molecular Medical Science Series

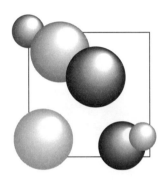

Molecular Aspects of Dermatology

Edited by
G. C. PRIESTLEY
Department of Dermatology, The University of Edinburgh, UK

JOHN WILEY & SONS
Chichester · New York · Brisbane · Toronto · Singapore

Other Wiley Editorial Offices

John Wiley & Sons, Inc., 605 Third Avenue,
New York, NY 10158–0012, USA

Jacaranda Wiley Ltd, G.P.O. Box 859, Brisbane,
Queensland 4001, Australia

John Wiley & Sons (Canada) Ltd, 22 Worcester Road,
Rexdale, Ontario M9W 1L1, Canada

John Wiley & Sons (SEA) Pte Ltd, 37 Jalan Pemimpin #05–04,
Block B, Union Industrial Building, Singapore 2057

Library of Congress Cataloging-in-Publication Data

Molecular aspects of dermatology / edited by G. C. Priestley.
    p.   cm.
    Includes bibliographical references and index.
    ISBN 0 471 93639 1
    1. Skin—Diseases—Molecular aspects.   2. Skin—Molecular aspects.
I. Priestley, G. C. (Graham C.)
    [DNLM: 1. Skin Diseases—genetics.   2. Skin—cytology.   WR 101
M7176 1993]
RL96.M65   1993
616.5'071—dc20
DNLM/DCL
for Library of Congress   93-2652
                                                                      CIP

British Library Cataloguing in Publication Data

A catalogue record for this book is available from the British Library

ISBN 0 471 93639 1

Typeset in 11/12pt Palatino by Vision Typesetting, Manchester
Printed and bound in Great Britain by Biddles Ltd, Guildford

Contents

Contributors

Paul E. Bowden
Department of Dermatology, University of Wales College of Medicine, Heath Park, Cardiff CF4 4XN, UK

Michael J. Cork
Sections of Dermatology and Molecular Medicine, Department of Medicine, University of Sheffield, Royal Hallamshire Hospital, Glossop Road, Sheffield S10 2JF, UK

Peter Critchley
Unilever Research Laboratories, Colworth House, Sharnbrook, Bedford MK44 1LQ, UK

Gordon W. Duff
Sections of Dermatology and Molecular Medicine, Department of Medicine, University of Sheffield, Royal Hallamshire Hospital, Glossop Road, Sheffield S10 2JF, UK

Michael Edward
Department of Dermatology, University of Glasgow, Robertson Building, 56 Dumbarton Road, Glasgow GU11 6NU, UK

John B. Mee
Sections of Dermatology and Molecular Medicine, Department of Medicine, University of Sheffield, Royal Hallamshire Hospital, Glossop Road, Sheffield S10 2JF, UK

Graham C. Priestley
Department of Dermatology, University of Edinburgh, Lauriston Building, The Royal Infirmary, Edinburgh EH3 9YW, UK

Jonathan L. Rees
Department of Dermatology, University of Newcastle upon Tyne, Royal Victoria Infirmary, Newcastle NE1 4LP, UK

Braham Shroot
CIRD Galderma, 635 Route des Lucioles, Sophia Antipolis, F-06565 Valbonne, France

A.J. Thody
Department of Dermatology, University of Newcastle upon Tyne, Royal Victoria Infirmary, Newcastle upon Tyne NE1 4LP, UK

Michael J. Tidman
Department of Dermatology, University of Edinburgh Lauriston Building, The Royal Infirmary, Edinburgh EH3 9YW, UK

Jacqueline B. Weiss
Department of Rheumatology, Wolfson Angiogenesis Unit, University of Manchester, Clinical Sciences Building, Hope Hospital, Salford M6 8HD, UK

Preface

The skin is the largest and most visible organ in the body. When we consider its diverse appearances among different mammals and take into account the activities of its hair follicles and glands, it becomes the original Amazing Technicolor Dream Coat. It offers protection against a hostile environment, (almost) never wears out, adapts to changing conditions, heals after injury, and does it all with style!

Although readily accessible for study, many of the skin's mysteries are only now being solved and dermatologists have adequate answers for disappointingly few of its confusing catalogue of over 2000 human skin disorders. Cutaneous diseases remain a major cause of embarrassment, discomfort and incapacity and are responsible for huge costs in health care and loss of working days. Surveys of British and North American communities have suggested that 23% and 31% respectively of the adult populations have skin disease severe enough to justify medical care (though many of those surveyed had not consulted a doctor) and there is evidence of a rising prevalence of some diseases.

Fortunately our knowledge of the basic biology and biochemistry of the skin is now expanding rapidly. Refinements in cell culture and the application of improved two-dimensional electrophoresis and new batteries of monoclonal antibodies have confirmed that the major skin proteins keratin and collagen belong to complex families of related molecules, which may be present in different combinations in different sites and different circumstances. A similar degree of complexity is also emerging for the proteoglycans, which were previously regarded as no more than inert structural elements of connective tissues. Cutaneous cells are now recognised as both a source of and a target for a whole range of mediators, making the skin part of the immune system. As research into many skin diseases begins to move from the protein to the DNA level, and the histopathologists, biochemists and immunologists are increasingly joined in the laboratory by molecular geneticists, this is a particularly exciting time to look at the skin and its wide range of molecules in the company of a band of expert guides.

Graham Priestley

1 An Introduction to the Skin and its Diseases

GRAHAM C. PRIESTLEY

The title of this monograph, *Molecular Aspects of Dermatology*, should not be read in the limited sense of molecular biology for clinical dermatologists. Dermatology, the study of the skin and its appendages, plays a part in the work of many other people, including plastic surgeons, veterinary surgeons, textile technologists, microbiologists, and cell biologists, while many tissue culturists grow skin fibroblasts or keratinocytes in their laboratories. We are primarily concerned with the *human* skin, but we hope that all these people will find something interesting here. In this first chapter the scene is set and some of the terms and structures which will be mentioned later by the specialist authors are introduced.

Our skin seems extremely familiar to us. We claim to know things 'like the back of our hand' and we inspect our faces daily in the mirror when shaving or applying cosmetics. Yet the familiarity is deceptive. Some regions of our skin are out of sight of all but a double-jointed mirror fetishist and there is a lot of it: an adult man has about 2 m² of skin surface, with marked regional variation and millions of hairs and glands. Look, for a moment, at the two surfaces of your hand. The marked contrasts in hairiness, surface topography and skin thickness show the skin to be far from the uniform sheet it appears at first sight; and many of its mysteries are only now beginning to be solved.

KERATIN AND KERATINOCYTES

Central among such puzzles is the nature of keratin. If the skin is principally a protective garment, insulating our sensitive inner tissues from the harsh environment, and its outer substance is composed of dead and hardened epithelial cells in a 'horny layer', then the chemistry of this hard material is crucial to our understanding of skin function.

The early microscopists took the name *keratin* from the Greek *keratos*, for horn, and the skin surface clearly has something in common with other hardened epithelial structures such as horn, hoof, claw, nail, hair and feather.

Molecular Aspects of Dermatology. Edited by G.C. Priestley.
© 1993 by John Wiley & Sons Ltd

The question then arose as to whether the keratin of these diverse structures was a single protein, perhaps modified for each different site, or whether there was more than one keratin. The wool chemists of Yorkshire and Australia soon appreciated that the hardness, insolubility and strength of keratin was due to disulphide bonds between and within its long-chain molecules of fibrous protein. By the early 1960s it was known that the sulphur-containing amino acids cysteine and methionine were incorporated into wool and hair follicles at a relatively late stage, that is, higher up the follicle than the bulb where the presumptive hair cortex cells were generated. Studies of skin had shown a similar two-stage incorporation. Did this indicate synthesis of a sulphur-rich protein which was added to the keratin protein already present in the cells?

The first electron micrographs of mature hairs showed fibrous elements – microfibrils – embedded in an electron-dense matrix, the staining properties of which suggested a high content of sulphur. This was enough to convince many investigators that hair was composed of a fibrous keratin, in these microfibrils, surrounded by at least one sulphur-containing amorphous keratin in the matrix. Combinations of the same two proteins in different proportions would explain the failure to obtain a consistent amino acid composition in hair and wool, and at once demolish the concept of keratin as a 'junk protein' of no fixed amino acid composition.

Thirty years later, safe in the now elementary knowledge that proteins have specific amino acid sequences dictated by messenger RNA and ultimately by DNA, the very idea of junk proteins seems quaint. Electrophoresis of epidermal keratins on polyacrylamide gels has shown a range of proteins with molecular weights in the range 40–70 kDa. We can now map the distribution of each molecule in a tissue using monoclonal antibodies and confirm that there may be up to a dozen different keratins in the epidermis and even more in the hair cortex. Their story is explained by Paul Bowden in Chapter 2.

The reason for introducing the keratins here at such length is twofold. First, their nature is fundamental to the protective functioning of the skin, and second, early attempts to understand the 'biomolecular structure' of keratin were a stepping stone in the pathway towards the unravelling of the structure of DNA itself. Astbury's first X-ray diffraction pictures of wool encouraged Crick and others to pursue the crystallographic technique with DNA, and Astbury was known to use the phrase 'molecular biology' in his laboratory at Leeds before it came into general currency.

The mixture of keratins in the horny layer provides a superbly adapted covering for the underlying tissues, being chemically unreactive, hard and waterproof (in both directions), yet elastic and resistant to abrasion and physical insult. The epithelial cells which produce keratin make up the bulk of the epidermis – more than 85% of its cell mass (Fig. 1.1) – and are called *keratinocytes*. They have been graphically, if crudely, defined as cells which produce so much keratin that they eventually choke themselves to death with it. Keratinocytes certainly specialise in making keratins, but are less completely dedicated to keratin synthesis than was previously thought. The amazing range of proteins they can produce is illustrated in Fig. 1.2.

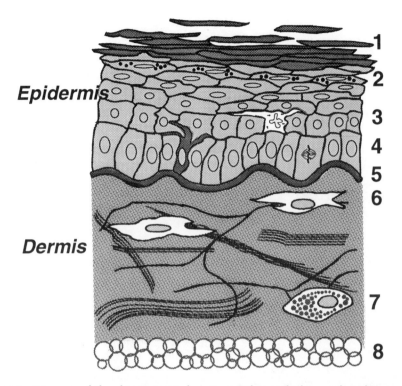

Fig. 1.1. Diagram of the skin in vertical section. Relative thickness of epidermis and dermis varies, but the dermis is usually thicker than shown here and blood vessels have been omitted from it for clarity. (1) Horny layer shedding dead corneocytes; (2) granular layer; (3) prickle cell layers with Langerhans cell (white) among the keratinocytes; (4) basal layer with melanocyte (dark) and one keratinocyte in mitosis; (5) basement membrane; (6) fibroblasts in the upper dermis among the collagen bundles, elastic fibres (branched) and glycosaminoglycans (grey background); (7) mast cell in the lower dermis; (8) subdermal fat

EPIDERMAL CELL PROLIFERATION AND DIFFERENTIATION

Keratinocytes are generated by mitoses in the *basal layer** of the epidermis and pass outwards through successive stages of differentiation towards the skin surface, where they are shed. Keratinocytes next become *spinous or prickle cells*, so called from the tiny points of intercellular contact, the *desmosomes*, which function like spot welds between adjacent cells. There are usually several layers of spinous cells below the *granular layer*. Here the cells contain large granules grouped round the nuclei and composed of a material named *keratohyalin* by the early microscopists, who regarded it as a soluble precursor of the insoluble

---

*The English names for epidermal cell layers will be used throughout this book instead of their Latin equivalents. Hence the *basal layer* corresponds to the stratum basale (or stratum germinativum), the *spinous or prickle cell layer* to the stratum spinosum, the *granular layer* to the stratum granulosum, and the *horny layer* to the stratum corneum.

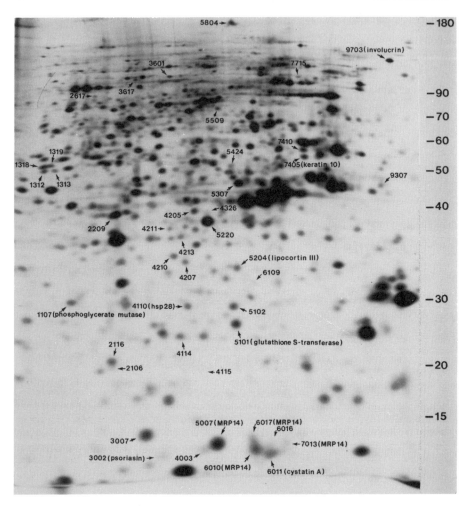

Fig. 1.2. Two-dimensional map of proteins synthesised by normal human epidermal keratinocytes. The spots represent radioactively labelled proteins separated on a polyacrylamide gel, first by electrofocusing (from left to right) and then by electrophoresis (from top to bottom) and detected on X-ray film following fluorography to increase sensitivity. Molecular weights (kDa) are indicated on the right and reference numbers were assigned as part of a standard database. A total of 2651 cellular proteins were resolved, of which 207 were identified. Reproduced from Celis *et al.* (1991) by kind permission of VCH Verlagsgesellschaft mbH

keratin of the *horny layer*. Hyalin(e) is the histologists' word for clear and the keratohyalin looks like clear droplets when stained with haematoxylin and viewed by light microscopy. The first electron micrographs of skin showed filaments of keratin in all layers of the epidermis, and disproved the idea that keratohyalin was the sole precursor of the material in the horny layer. Keratohyalin remained an intriguing puzzle for many years but is now thought to contribute several proteins, notably the histidine-rich protein filaggrin, to the final mixture present in the dead cells.

The transition from living granular layer to dead horny layer is abrupt and the granular layer is usually only one or two cells thick. The horny layer, in contrast, is usually many cells thick, reaching impressive dimensions (up to 600 μm) on the palm and sole. It provides the main protective barrier of the skin, and prevents 98% of the water loss which would occur through an open wound. If it is stripped off with Sellotape, as an experimental procedure, water loss becomes uncontrolled, penetration of drugs is greatly increased and there is an immediate danger of infection. It appears to be the dryness of the normal skin surface which makes it an inhospitable home for microorganisms: they can survive there, but only flourish when the horny surface is damaged and hydrated by disease or by impermeable dressings.

The control of mitosis and epidermal cell production is another fascinating problem. Our skin fits us well, although it grows somewhat baggy in our later years. A control mechanism must operate, therefore, in normal skin, which is overridden to allow repair in a healing wound. In hyperproliferative diseases, like psoriasis, this control is defective. The over-production of cells is seen as the shedding of skin scales, which is most obvious on the elbows and knees. Up to one million people in the UK alone suffer from psoriasis, which causes social misery and physical incapacity in the most severe cases. It is a major medical problem, taking up many hospital beds, out-patient facilities and much general practitioner time.

A massive world-wide research effort has failed to find the cause of psoriasis and of its central feature, epidermal hyperproliferation, but we now understand more about the basic mechanisms at work (Mier and van der Kerkof, 1986). We know that in normal skin almost half the cells in the basal layer are outside the cell cycle and therefore do not divide. These quiescent cells can be recruited into the cycle in an emergency, for instance to repair a wound. The emergency procedure is also activated in the lesions of psoriasis, so that all the basal cells there cycle and divide. But what switches on this recruitment, and what prevents it in normal skin? There have been many suggestions over the years, including hormones, enzymes, cyclic nucleotides, prostaglandins, metal ions, and tissue-specific mitotic inhibitors termed *chalones*, but the most attractive theory today is that there is an imbalance of inhibitory and stimulatory *cytokines*.

These are low-molecular-weight mediators, by which cells communicate and influence one another's activities. Unlike the chalones, which remain a hypothetical concept, many cytokines have been identified and characterised and the psoriatic keratinocyte may well be the slave of some other cell. Both lymphocytes and dermal fibroblasts have been suggested for this role. One of the first cytokines to be described was interleukin 1 (IL-1), which was first regarded as a product of macrophages, but later found to be secreted by keratinocytes themselves. Many more interleukins and other cytokines are now known and because they may interact and some cells may be both sources and targets, the possibilities for complicated control mechanisms are numerous. Michael Cork, John Mee and Gordon Duff keep us up to date with this challenging and constantly developing topic in Chapter 7.

SKIN PIGMENTATION

The skin has several other functions besides being a physical barrier (Table 1.1). Dermatologists may be less aware than zoologists of the role of pigments in camouflage and predator–prey relationships, but dermatology departments now see increasing numbers of patients worried about pigmented lesions and possible skin cancer, as well as a few with failures of skin pigmentation such as vitiligo or albinism. The colour of our skin is a complex blend in which the brown pigment *melanin* is one of the main ingredients. Skin colour is one way in which we communicate; most obviously by blushing or pallor, but the texture, tone and degree of tanning of our skin, and the colour and amount of the hair it bears, all contribute to our identity and our sexual image, as perceived by ourselves and by others.

Ultraviolet radiation can damage or even kill unprotected cells. Although some of its rays are reflected from the surface of the horny layer and more are

Table 1.1. Functions and properties of the skin

1. *Protects* against:
   physical and chemical trauma
   penetration of chemicals and drugs
   water loss (and entry)
   ultraviolet radiation
   infection

2. *Provides sensory information* (hot, cold, sharp, smooth)

3. *Insulates* and provides special mechanisms for temperature control (vasodilation and vasoconstriction; evaporative sweating)

4. *Synthesises* vitamin D

5. *Provides containment* for internal organs (made effective by elasticity)

6. *Contributes to our physical and sexual identity* through its colour, texture and amount of hair it bears

7. *Has some communication functions* (as 6 above) and through blushing, pallor and sweating. May provide an indicator of internal disease

8. *Secretes* sweat and sebum. Apocrine glands, largely vestigial in humans, *may secrete pheromones*

9. *Adapts* in response to stimuli and is self-regenerating and self-healing

absorbed by its dense protein mass, melanin pigments, concentrated in oval granules called *melanosomes*, absorb radiation at the most dangerous wavelengths (290–320 μm) and shield the keratinocyte nuclei and their DNA. Melanosomes are produced in epidermal pigment cells (*melanocytes*) in the basal layer of the epidermis and the hair follicle bulb. Each melanocyte transfers melanin to a clutch of about 30 surrounding keratinocytes through long processes called dendrites. The familiar brown-black pigment is sometimes referred to as *eumelanin*, to distinguish it from *phaeomelanin*, which is yellow-red. Tony Thody, whose laboratory at Newcastle recently confirmed the presence of phaeomelanin in skin (it was well known already in hair), describes the melanins and other skin pigments in Chapter 3.

OTHER EPIDERMAL CELL TYPES

In addition to the keratinocytes and melanocytes, the epidermis contains two further cell types: the *Langerhans* and *Merkel* cells. Paul Langerhans discovered the cell that now bears his name just over 100 years ago. The Langerhans cell is another dendritic cell, which lacks keratin filaments and pigment granules. It occurs in the suprabasal epidermis among the lower spinous cells (Fig. 1.1) and was regarded as a curiosity, possibly a worn-out melanocyte, for many years. The discovery in the 1950s by electron microscopy of unique tennis racket-shaped granules in sections of Langerhans cell cytoplasm indicated a different lineage. We now know that Langerhans cells are antigen-presenting cells which originate in the bone marrow. They behave like epidermal macrophages in their capacity to present antigen to T-lymphocytes but lack the phagocytic capacity of macrophages.

Langerhans cells are a source of cytokines, especially IL-1. They bear class II major histocompatibility complex antigens (HLA-DR, -DP and -DQ). They take part in the immunosurveillance of viral and tumour antigens and their damage by ultraviolet light may be an important part of the pathway to some skin cancers.

Merkel cells are non-dendritic cells lying in or near the basal layer in association with hair follicles. They act as transducers for touch and fine unmyelinated nerve endings are often associated with them.

THE BASEMENT MEMBRANE

All epithelia have a basement membrane. In the skin this thin layer, sometimes referred to as the junctional zone, separates and holds together the epidermis and the dermis. Although it can be recognised with light microscopy using special histochemical procedures (periodic acid–Schiff or silver impregnation), the basement membrane was first characterised by electron microscopy and the names of its two layers relate to this history. Immediately below the epidermal basal cells is the *lamina lucida*, a zone which looks clear in the electron beam. Beneath this is the *lamina densa*, which stains more heavily and looks opaque.

The first components of the basement membrane to be identified included the glycoproteins *laminin, type IV collagen* and *bullous pemphigoid antigen*. The use of monoclonal antibodies is revealing many more. *Fibronectin, type V collagen* and *thrombospondin* may be associated with the basement membrane zone but are not structural components. Other membrane structures are concerned with anchorage. The basal surface of the keratinocytes bears *hemidesmosomes* which attach them to the lamina lucida. The lamina densa is traversed by fine *anchoring fibrils* which are composed of type VII collagen and terminate in the dermis, possibly in irregular electron-dense bodies called *anchoring plaques*. Deficiencies in these anchoring structures, which may be genetically determined or acquired, permit the junctional zone to break down, a process leading to the formation of a blister. In fact blistering can develop, above, within and below the basement membrane, so that the diagnosis of the many blistering (or *bullous*) conditions is a complex clinical problem, requiring electron microscopy and the use of antibodies directed against specific components of the basement membrane. Mike Tidman describes the molecular make-up of the basement membrane zone in Chapter 4.

THE DERMIS

For many years the dermis was regarded as a relatively inert support for the epidermis. The sparseness of the cells lurking among the fibres in the adult dermis seemed to confirm that impression, and there was also evidence that the collagen fibres of the rat dermis lasted for the animal's entire lifetime. We now appreciate, however, that the dermis has a complex metabolism and may influence the embryonic development, and to some extent the later functioning, of the epidermis. If keratins are regarded as the first family of skin proteins, then collagens are the second. Yet Jackie Weiss, who writes on collagens and other dermal proteins in Chapter 6, might want to reverse that order of importance. She could make a strong case: collagen accounts for 70% of the skin's fat-free dry weight in humans and is one of the most ubiquitous proteins in the animal kingdom. The commercial importance of leather and the ease with which human joints are damaged have helped to make collagen one of the most investigated of all proteins. Indeed our awareness of collagens as a family of molecules came before we knew about the family of keratins. The number of collagen types, currently 14, is constantly expanding. In the skin about 80% of the collagen is type I, with 15% of type III. Only small amounts of other collagens are present, but some are arranged in the critically important structures of the basement membrane (types IV and VII).

A simple low-power view of the dermis in a section stained with haemotoxylin and eosin shows masses of red-stained collagen bundles occupying virtually the entire space. The cells that lie among the fibres, and were from the earliest days assumed to produce them, are called *fibroblasts* (a fashion for 'fibrocytes' has declined). The ease with which fibroblasts can be cultured from skin (Fig. 1.3) and other connective tissues, and maintained for long periods *in vitro*, has made them extremely familiar, sometimes as a convenient model for a generalised cell rather than for their own sake. For almost 50 years cultured fibroblasts were regarded as dedifferentiated, like the cells of embryonic tissue, but that changed in the 1960s when cultured fibroblasts were found to synthesise both collagen and glycosaminoglycans, the amorphous ground substance of the dermis (Green and Hamerman, 1964).

The histologists had also demonstrated a second system of fibres in the dermis, the elastic fibre network. This contributes extensibility and contractility to the tissue, but it was another 20 years before it was proved that elastin, which with the microfibrillar protein goes to make up the elastic fibres, was also a fibroblast product (Giro *et al.*, 1985). It is now appreciated that fibroblasts also control the turnover of connective tissue by producing enzymes which degrade collagens (collagenases), elastin (elastase), proteoglycans and glycosaminoglycans (stromelysin and lysosomal hydrolases). The ageing of connective tissue, with its loss of strength and elasticity, and impaired healing of wounds, is therefore another problem which can be studied using cultured fibroblasts. Synthesis of dermal macromolecules and their degradative enzymes can be compared in fibroblast lines derived from people of various ages.

Many connective tissue abnormalities are expressed *in vitro* and cultured skin fibroblasts have been used in the diagnosis of certain inherited skin diseases. An example is the group of mucopolysaccharide (glycosaminoglycan) storage diseases, where the enzymes which degrade these relatively short-lived carbohydrate polymers are deficient. In the normal skin, glycosaminoglycans are responsible for binding water, and this controls the tone and turgor of the tissue and helps to resist compression. In fact, glycosaminoglycans are present in only small amounts, accounting for about 0.1% of the dry weight of the skin, but, remarkably, they can bind over one hundred times their own weight of water. Mike Edward tells us more about glycosaminoglycans and proteoglycans in Chapter 5.

The second cell type of the dermis is the *mast cell*, characterised by its large cytoplasmic granules. These were originally thought to be nutrient stores but in fact contain histamine, enzymes and other mediators which are discharged as part of the inflammatory response. Mast cells bind immunoglobulin E (IgE), high levels of which are a central feature of the allergies which plague many patients attending dermatology clinics.

The cells and extracellular material of the dermis account for its substance, but it also contains, or is traversed by, blood vessels, nerves and pilosebaceous units (the hair follicles with their associated muscle and glands).

The blood vessels lie in two main horizontal layers with vertical connections and terminate in fine capillary networks just beneath the epidermis. There are no blood vessels in the epidermis, nutrients required by the epidermal cells and any cellular waste products having to pass through the capillary walls and the basement membrane. Constriction and dilation of the vessels are important in the control of skin (and body) temperature. Venous insufficiency, especially in middle-aged women, is one cause of a major dermatological problem, the leg ulcer. As ulcers may take months to heal, the cost of treating them in hospital wards is considerable. New synthetic dressings, for example hydrocolloids, which discourage microbial growth and seem to promote healing, promise more successful and cost-effective treatment for the patient at home (Robinson, 1988).

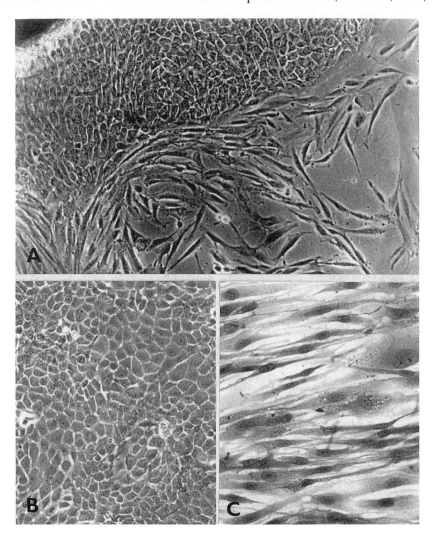

The sensations of pain and itch help to protect the skin and itching is also a symptom of many skin diseases; indeed in pruritus the itch is sometimes regarded as the disease itself. The skin is richly supplied with nerve endings, some of which are free and respond to heat and trauma. Others terminate in Merkel cells or special end organs such as Paccinian and Meissner corpuscles, which are mechanoreceptors and lie just beneath the epidermis.

HAIR FOLLICLES AND GLANDS

Hair follicles, sweat and sebaceous glands are epidermal structures (Fig. 1.4) and grow down into the embryonic dermis. The sebaceous glands secrete their sebum into the neck of the follicle close to the skin surface. Apocrine sweat glands are restricted to axillary, anogenital and nipple areas and their secretion too is discharged into the follicle lumen. Eccrine sweat glands, in contrast, are found all over the body unassociated with hair follicles: they discharge directly onto the surface. Each eccrine gland is a single unbranched tube, coiled into a ball-like mass deep in the dermis and then serving as its own duct as it rises towards the skin surface. The eccrine glands are particularly numerous on the palms, soles ($620/cm^2$) and forehead ($360/cm^2$) skin. They are responsible for evaporative cooling by the continuous secretion of about 0.5 litres of sweat per day in an adult, but can reach ten times that rate of production in severe heat stress. Eccrine sweat is more than 99% water, with traces of lactic acid, amino acids, urea, salts, proteins and nucleic acid. The apocrine sweat appears to be a vestigial product in man, but is responsible for body odour following the action of bacteria and may contain pheromones – the odoriferous secretions known to influence the behaviour of other animals within the same species. There is only

---

Fig. 1.3. Cell cultures derived from skin. A: Primary culture with keratinocytes and fibroblasts growing out from an explant of skin. Phase-contrast; × 156. B: Secondary culture of keratinocytes. Phase-contrast; × 228. C: Secondary culture of fibroblasts. Giemsa-stained; × 293. It is also possible to isolate melanocytes in pure culture. Studies of such monolayer cultures (cells growing as a thin carpet on the bottom of a plastic dish or flask) have greatly enhanced knowledge of normal and abnormal skin. Advantages over whole skin include: a controlled environment for growth; ready availability of enough material (perhaps from a named patient or condition) for biochemical analysis; direct viewing by phase-contrast microscopy of living cells of a single type; and accurate quantification by electronic cell counting or DNA analysis. The last point is important for a tissue where variations in thickness complicate the use of wet weight, and the elasticity of the skin complicates use of surface area as indices. Important areas of use have been keratin expression, collagen synthesis, drug toxicity and pharmacology, disease pathogenesis, and provision of keratinocyte grafts for patients with severe burns or leg ulcers. Direct effects of drugs on a particular cell have been demonstrated in the absence of blood vessels, nerves or other cell types, often for the first time, and many novel actions of drugs have been discovered. Recent developments include fibroblast culture in three-dimensional collagen lattices to provide a more dermally realistic system and co-culture of the lattices with keratinocytes to study epithelial–mesenchymal interaction

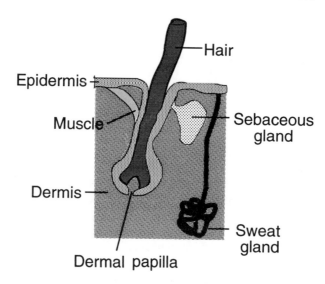

Hair

Epidermis

Muscle

Sebaceous gland

Dermis

Sweat gland

Dermal papilla

Fig. 1.4. Diagram of a pilosebaceous unit (hair follicle group) in the active (anagen) phase of the hair growth cycle. An eccrine sweat gland and duct are shown on the right

indirect evidence for the existence of human pheromones.

The sebaceous glands are extremely active and well developed in many mammals. In the merino sheep, for instance, almost half the weight of the fleece can be wool grease secreted by sebaceous glands. The coats of carnivores owe something of their sleekness to sebum and to constant grooming. Human sebaceous glands are largely vestigial; the fact that they are barely functional before puberty points to our lack of reliance on them, although as the skin's most obvious source of lipid they were suspected of providing a waterproof surface to the horny layer. In fact epidermal cells synthesise a wide range of lipids of their own (described by Peter Critchley in Chapter 8), the presence of which is sufficient to explain the waterproofing, which fails only when the whole horny layer is removed.

Another possible role for sebum relates to its free fatty acids, released from triglycerides by bacterial lipases. Some fatty acids are antimicrobial *in vitro*, which prompted the suggestion that they could provide a self-sterilising capability for the skin. This idea now seems rather fanciful in view of the small quantities of sebum present on the skin and its low content of those acids with antimicrobial potential. It is more likely that the very dryness of the normal skin surface discourages the growth of microorganisms. A mixture of yeasts, micrococci and bacilli inhabits the surface, and the ducts of the glands and follicles, but cannot flourish unless the horny layer is hydrated or damaged.

Another problem which relates to sebum production is acne. The amount of sebum a person produces, that is, the sebum secretion rate, usually measured on the forehead, may influence the severity of any acne that will develop.

Consequently much acne therapy is aimed at reducing sebaceous secretion. Systemic treatment with the retinoid isotretinoin, (13-*cis*-retinoic acid), for example, is an option for patients with severe and chronic acne. Such treatment can damage the sebaceous glands, without any apparent effect on the rate of water loss or skin microflora, another indication that their function is not essential.

Both sebum secretion and hair growth are highly androgen dependent. Two more unsolved cutaneous mysteries are why acne improves after the teenage years when hormone levels and sebum secretion are relatively stable, and how androgens can promote increased hair growth via follicle enlargement at puberty and yet later be involved in male pattern baldness, that is, in the progressive regression of certain scalp hair follicles.

The hair follicle itself is a highly differentiated structure (Fig. 1.4). It is a tube open at one end onto the skin surface and blind at the other, where it swells into a bulbous shape like an onion. The epithelium of the follicle bulb is closely associated with a plug of specialised dermis containing cells and blood vessels, the *dermal papilla*, which in some way regulates the cycle of activity in the follicle. An active phase, *anagen*, in which a hair is produced, is followed by a quiescent phase, *telogen*. The duration of anagen determines the final length of the hair, and is a characteristic of any particular body region. Anagen in scalp and beard follicles may last 3–6 years, but is a matter of only weeks or months elsewhere on the body. Human scalp hair grows at about 0.33 mm per day, or 1 cm per month, which is far slower than some animal hairs. The guard hairs of the rat and wool on Wensleydale sheep, for example, may exceed 1 mm per day.

SKIN DISEASE: ITS PREVALENCE AND COST

Medical students are impressed and perhaps depressed when told that there are some 2000 different diseases of the skin. Two questions they often ask are 'What are the most *common* skin diseases?' and 'Which are the most *serious* skin diseases?' But the simple answers they expect are elusive. Estimates of the commonness of any skin disease, that is, its prevalence or the number of cases per 10 000 population at a single point in time, depend on who is making the assessment and where. Surveys of the population as a whole are rare, although one was made in Lambeth, London, in 1976. Cases seen by general practitioners are better documented but are an unrepresentative sample because many people are ignorant of their condition or treat it themselves, with or without the aid of their local pharmacist. The cases referred by general practitioners to dermatologist specialists in the UK are fewer still (representing perhaps 3% of the original total) and different again, but are the best documented.

Even in the UK, therefore, we have three types of data. The Lambeth community survey (Rae *et al.*, 1976) included over 2000 adults and found an overall prevalence of 22.5% for skin disease severe enough to justify medical care. Within this percentage only one-fifth had consulted a doctor; the most common condition was eczema (6%). A much larger survey in the USA (the Health And National Examination Survey, 1978) found an overall prevalence of 31% in the general population, with diseases of sebaceous glands (mainly acne) as the most common condition. We should expect differences in prevalence between different countries, reflecting climate, social habits and conditions, ethnic background and the age structure of the population. Third World countries have more infectious disease, Australasia and the USA more skin cancer, young populations have more acne and older populations more senile keratoses and shingles.

A survey of 48 British general practices representing 332 270 patients in 1981–82 showed an increased rate of consultation for skin complaints compared to 1955–56. Viral warts, atopic eczema and acne were the largest groups. Attempts to define changes in the prevalence of disease are full of pitfalls, but a recent analysis of the data for atopic dermatitis (which include claims of two- to fivefold rises over 30 years) concluded that there had indeed been a real increase in prevalence in recent years (Williams, 1992). Table 1.2 gives a breakdown of the most frequent diagnoses from 20 252 visits to American dermatologists' office practices: sebaceous disorders are well ahead of the rest, with eczema/dermatitis in second place.

In Britain the most serious conditions will be those seen by dermatologists in hospitals. The data from our Edinburgh Department (Harris *et al.*, 1990) are probably fairly representative in showing a rising tide of pigmented lesions (only a few of which turn out to be malignant melanomas) and dermatitis, set against steadier flows of patients with, for example, psoriasis and leg ulcers. The relative 'seriousness' of these conditions is open to debate: is a small

Table 1.2. Most frequent dermatological diagnoses in office practices in the USA

Diagnosis	% of total	Mean age	Sex (% male)
1. Sebaceous gland disorders (acne)	20	22	34
2. Eczema and dermatitis	15	40	40
3. Viral diseases (warts and herpes)	7	24	46
4. Malignant neoplasms (melanoma)	6	63	55
5. Hypertrophies/atrophies	5	58	51
6. Psoriasis	5	42	45
7. Benign neoplasms (moles)	4	52	39
8. Hair diseases	2	34	44
9. Fungal infections	2	36	52
10. Congenital abnormalities	2	32	35
11. Pruritus (itching)	2	47	40
12. Erythematous conditions (red skin)	2	47	34

Adapted from Johnson *et al.* (1979).

pigmented lesion which might be a melanoma and therefore might carry a finite risk of death, more serious than a recurrent leg ulcer which keeps the patient in hospital for several months? The very visibility of skin diseases, and other people's reactions to them (especially an unwarranted fear of infection), are important components of their seriousness which don't apply to heart or kidney disease. Two indices of seriousness are mortality and cost. Fortunately, skin diseases kill relatively few people (0.5% of all deaths in the USA): melanomas and other malignancies are the largest category. In terms of cost, skin conditions came second to repeated trauma as the greatest cause of lost working days in the USA (1975 figures). The annual cost of drugs used to treat the skin is now estimated at £100 million in Britain, but this figure is too low because treatments with general drugs, like antibiotics, cannot be identified and are excluded.

INHERITANCE OF SKIN DISEASE

Many skin diseases are inherited. In some, an obvious pattern of, for example, autosomal dominant inheritance was almost the only well-understood feature of the condition. Autosomal recessive inheritance is seen in many of the rare skin diseases. There are also some where a familial pattern is obvious but imprecise, examples being psoriasis and vitiligo, and geneticists use terms like *incomplete penetrance* or *multifactorial inheritance* in explanation. Molecular genetics has provided techniques whereby genes can be mapped to a particular chromosome, sequenced and, perhaps ultimately, replaced. There have been some spectacular successes, for instance in muscular dystrophy, and we can expect many more. For some diseases, however, prenatal diagnosis is the most encouraging practical advance for the parents at risk, providing them with the chance to have a healthy child. Jonathan Rees writes on the molecular genetics of the skin in Chapter 9.

DRUGS FOR THE SKIN

Until genetic correction is possible, those who have the 'wrong' genes must rely mainly on therapy with drugs for control of their disease. Physiotherapy, irradiation and minor surgery also have their place in the dermatologist's armoury, as do preventative techniques in appropriate conditions.

The scientist new to dermatology would like to believe that a new therapy should evolve along logical lines. Adequate research should discover the cause and mechanism of the disease process and pharmacology would then provide a 'golden bullet', to correct the defect without causing other problems. Unfortunately there are difficulties with every stage of this scenario. Research is seldom adequately funded and its progress is unpredictable: for example, the huge effort to explain psoriasis has had only limited success. Next the selection of a drug for a specific task assumes that we have a vast array of drugs and completely understand their capabilities. Finally, the 'golden bullet' concept of striking a single target without side-effects is a dream. All drugs have a range of actions, some useful and some unpleasant or harmful (Albert, 1985). Many drugs nominated for a particular task have proved too toxic to be tolerated. As a result many conditions still lack an effective treatment.

This may sound depressingly negative, but progress can and is being made. It is worth mentioning an instance where the problem and its solution turned out to be relatively simple. In 1974 the London dermatologist Edmund Moynahan realised that *acrodermatitis enteropathica* was due to zinc deficiency (Moynahan, 1974). Its features included scaling and inflammation, particularly around the mouth and anus, loss of hair, and photophobia. The patients were depressed, with diarrhoea and little appetite. Until the mid-1970s the lives of the few survivors were ruined and the treatment available – oral administration of hydroxyquinolines – was difficult to tolerate. After Moynahan's insight, patients were given zinc sulphate tablets and their condition resolved in a few days. This is not a miracle cure: the patients must take the zinc supplements for the rest of their lives, but their disease is effectively controlled.

Solutions are seldom so simple. A more common experience is that of a drug which succeeds in one condition being tried for others and giving 'some benefit', which may or may not stand up to rigorous independent analysis. The logic for such open trials is that at worst they do no harm and might even bring improvement by a placebo effect. Such an approach is easy to mock but has had its successes. D-Penicillamine was introduced as a drug to break up immune complexes in rheumatoid arthritis. Instead it has found a place in the treatment of scleroderma for its ability to block the cross-linking of collagen, which accumulates in the thick and rigid skin.

The pharmaceutical industry has the means to generate thousands of compounds and then to select those with useful activity. The successful compounds then proceed to toxicity testing and later to clinical trials. It is a long and costly process: 1992 estimates are 12 years and £120 million per new drug from discovery to launch. Yet at its most successful the process can provide families of drugs in which the common molecular skeleton has been adapted to give a range of slightly different compounds. This may have two results: one is a series of drugs of gradually increasing potency but the same overall properties; the other is a series of drugs with different properties. The corticosteroids are a family of the first type. The basic cortisone and hydrocortisone molecules, which occur naturally in the body, were modified to provide other steroids with up to 2000 times the anti-inflammatory potency of hydrocortisone (according, at least, to the vasoconstrictor assay). Unfortunately, the greater potency brings with it an increase in side-effects. The retinoids – compounds related to vitamin A – are a family of the second type: different retinoids have different effects and, encouragingly, the

manufacturers can be confident that further exploration will yield still more useful compounds. Braham Shroot explains more about molecular pharmacology in Chapter 10.

REFERENCES

Albert A (1985) *Selective Toxicity*, 7th edn. London: Chapman & Hall.
Celis JE et al. (1991) Master 2D gel database of keratinocyte proteins. *Electrophoresis* **12**, 802–872.
Giro MG, Oikarinen AL, Oikarinen H, Sephel GC, Uitto J and Davidson JM (1985) Demonstration of elastin gene expression in human skin fibroblast cultures and reduced tropoelastin production from a patient with atrophoderma. *Journal of Clinical Investigation* **75**, 672–678.
Green H and Hamerman D (1964) Production of hyaluronate and collagen by fibroblast clones in culture. *Nature* **201**, 710.
Harris DWS, Benton EC and Hunter JAA (1990) The changing face of dermatology out-patient referrals in the south east of Scotland. *British Journal of Dermatology* **123**, 645–650.
Johnson M-LT, Burdick AE and Johnson KG (1979) Prevalence, morbidity and cost of dermatological disease. *Journal of Investigative Dermatology* **73**, 395–401.
Mier PD and van der Kerkof PCM (1986) *Textbook of Psoriasis*, p. 292. Edinburgh: Churchill Livingstone.
Moynahan EJ (1974) Acrodermatitis enteropathica, a lethal, inherited zinc-deficiency. *Lancet* **ii**, 399–400.
Rae JN, Newhouse ML and Halil T (1976) Skin disease in Lambeth: a community study of prevalence and use of medical care. *British Journal of Preventive and Social Medicine* **30**, 107–114.
Robinson BJ (1988) Randomised comparative study of Duoderm vs. viscopaste PB7 bandage in the management of venous leg ulceration and cost to the community. In: Ryan TJ (ed.) *Beyond Occlusion: Wound Care Proceedings*, pp. 101–104. Int. Congr. Symp. Series no. 136. London: Royal Society of Medicine.
Williams HC (1992) Is the prevalence of atopic dermatitis increasing? *Clinical and Experimental Dermatology* **17**, 385–391.

SUGGESTED FURTHER READING

Bereiter-Hahn J, Matoltsy AG and Richards KS (eds) (1984) *Biology of the Integument 2. Vertebrates*. Berlin: Springer-Verlag.
Champion RH, Burton J and Ebling FJG (eds) (1992) *Textbook of Dermatology*, 5th edn. London: Blackwell.
Hunter JAA, Savin JA and Dahl MV (1989) *Clinical Dermatology*. London: Blackwell.
Thody AJ and Friedman PS (eds) (1986) *Scientific Basis of Dermatology: A Physiological Approach*. Edinburgh: Churchill Livingstone.
Wood EJ and Bladon PT (1985) *The Human Skin*. London: Edward Arnold.

2 Keratins and Other Epidermal Proteins

PAUL E. BOWDEN

STRUCTURAL PROTEINS OF THE SKIN AND HAIR

Research over the last 20 years has greatly improved our knowledge of the structural proteins that form human skin and its appendages such as hair and nail. While the early work concentrated on characterising the physical properties of the skin and hair, some attempts were made to define the structural proteins themselves. The available experimental tools (histology, electron microscopy, X-ray diffraction, protein gel electrophoresis and isoelectric focusing, gel chromatography and amino acid analysis) allowed an initial characterisation of various skin proteins, but the picture obtained was often confusing and incomplete. However, significant advances in our understanding of many of these specialised structural proteins have been made in the last 10–15 years and much of the recent research has owed its success to the combined application of cell biology, biochemistry, immunology and molecular genetics. Particularly important in this respect has been the development of specific antisera to individual proteins, the cloning and manipulation of DNA (deoxyribonucleic acid) encoding skin structural proteins and the successful culture of various skin cell types (fibroblasts, keratinocytes and melanocytes).

The development of both polyclonal and monoclonal antisera to various skin structural proteins has helped to unravel the mysteries of their often complex expression, and has been particularly important for the understanding of a large multigene family of proteins such as the keratins. The availability of keratin antisera, and especially antisera that are monospecific for individual keratins, has been crucial to the study of keratin expression not only in the skin but also in other epithelial tissues (for review see Franke et al., 1982). Techniques such as immunohistochemistry, immunocytochemistry and immuno-gold electron microscopy have provided much information about keratin expression in epithelial tissues and have allowed views of the three-dimensional structure of the keratin intermediate filament (IF) network in epithelial cells (Fig. 2.1). Immunoblotting and immunoprecipitation, combined with polyacrylamide gel electrophoresis, have played an important role in the

Molecular Aspects of Dermatology. Edited of G.C. Priestley.
© 1993 by John Wiley & Sons Ltd

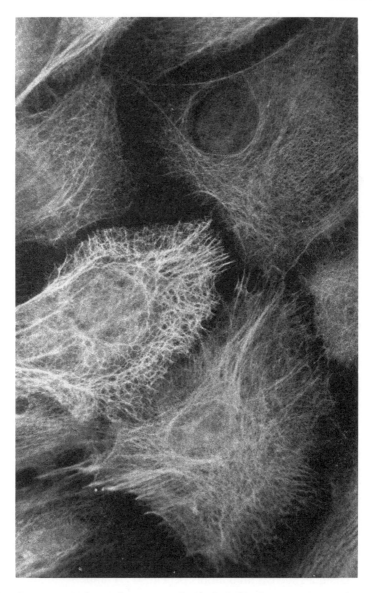

Fig. 2.1 Immunocytochemical staining of cultured skin keratinocytes with a specific antiserum to human keratins, demonstrating the three-dimensional network of keratin intermediate filaments that surround the nucleus and terminate at desmosomal junctions on the plasma membrane. Work done in collaboration with Prof. N.E. Fusenig, DKFZ, Heidelberg, Germany

characterisation of antisera, as these techniques reveal the specific size and charge properties of the antigens concerned. The skin is a complex and organised mixture of several cell types which form highly specialised structures (hair follicles and glands for example) and these methods have helped to tell us which cells synthesise and accumulate the many different keratins and the other major structural proteins of the skin and hair (Table 2.1).

Molecular genetic (or recombinant DNA) techniques, and the powerful combination of cell and molecular biology, have also contributed significantly to advances in the understanding of skin structural proteins and their genes. Over the last 10 years, it has been possible to isolate and characterise DNA clones (cDNA and genomic DNA) which encode many of the major structural proteins of the skin and hair. These include proteins that are specific to the epidermis and other skin epithelia (keratins, filaggrin, trichohyalin, loricrin and involucrin), the dermis (collagens, elastin, fibrillin, plectin and vimentin), the basement membrane zone (collagens, fibronectin, integrins, laminin, nicein, nidogen/entactin and thrombospondin) and the desmosome/hemidesmosome (desmoplakin, desmoglein, desmocollin and plakoglobin). The application of molecular biological techniques to these mostly very insoluble structural proteins has provided knowledge of their primary sequence and secondary structure which, at best, would have been technically extremely difficult to obtain by isolating and sequencing the proteins themselves. Furthermore, the isolation and sequencing of complete genes for some of these skin structural proteins have provided valuable information on gene structure (size, intron/exon boundaries) and has allowed more extensive studies of gene expression, gene localisation, gene regulation and the genetic basis of some skin diseases. For example, the chromosomal localisation of many skin genes has been identified by *in situ* hybridisation on metaphase chromosomes and by Southern blotting of somatic cell hybrid DNA with skin gene specific DNA probes

Table 2.1. Structural proteins of the skin and hair

Epidermis (keratinocyte)	Actin,[a] α-actinin, adducin, filaggrin, integrins,[b] involucrin, keratins (skin-specific),[c] loricrin, spectrin
Hair follicle	Keratins (skin-specific),[c] trichohyalin
Hair shaft/nail plate	Keratins (hair/nail-specific),[c] high and ultra-high-sulphur matrix proteins, high-glycine–tyrosine proteins
Intercellular junctions	Desmoplakin, desmoglein, desmocollin, cadherin, plakoglobin
Basement membrane zone	Collagens,[d] epiligrin, fibronectin, integrins,[b] laminin, nicein, nidogen (entactin), thrombospondin
Dermis (fibroblast)	Collagens,[g] elastin, fibrillin, integrins,[b] plectin, vimentin

[a]Actin is a ubiquitous cytoskeletal protein and present throughout the skin.
[b]About 22 integrins have been described (α1–8; αV, αL, αM, αX, αIIb, αHML-1; α1–8) and various heterodimers are expressed on epithelial cells (α2β1, α3β1, α6β1, α6β4, αVβ6), keratinocytes (α5β1) and fibroblasts (α6β4, αVβ1, αVβ3, αVβ5).
[c]About 30 keratins have been described (K1–K20, HaKb1–4, Hbx, HaKa1–4, Hax; members of IF multigene family) but they are not all expressed in skin, hair and nail.
[d]14 collagens have been described (types I, III, IV, VI, VII are common in skin).

Table 2.2. Chromosomal organisation of human skin structural genes

Chromosome 1	Collagen[a] (VIIIα2, XIα1), involucrin, laminin β2, loricrin, nidogen, profilaggrin, trichohyalin
Chromosome 2	Collagen (IIIα1, Vα2), integrin α6
Chromosome 3	Collagen (VIIIα1, XIα2, VII)
Chromosome 6	BP antigen,[b] collagen (Xα1, IXα1), desmoplakin (I, II)
Chromosome 7	Collagen (Iα2), desmoplakin (III), elastin, laminin β1
Chromosome 9	Desmoglein (II, III), tenascin[c]
Chromosome 10	Collagen (VIIIα1), fibronectin receptor β, vimentin, vinculin
Chromosome 12	Collagen (IIα1), keratins (type II)
Chromosome 13	Collagen (IVα1)
Chromosome 15	Fibrillin
Chromosome 17	Integrin β4, keratins (type I)
Chromosome 18	Desmoglein (I), laminin α
Chromosome 19	Fibronectin receptor α
Chromosome 21	Collagen (VIα1, VIα2)
Chromosome X	Collagen (IVα5)

[a]Collagen genes are spread throughout the genome. The major skin collagens are types I, III, IV, V, VI and VII.
[b]Bullous pemphigoid (BP) antigen is a component of the hemidesmosome.
[c]Tenascin is an integrin-related glycoprotein of the extracellular matrix.

(Table 2.2). This provides a good overview of the chromosomal organisation of skin structural proteins. Gene expression has been examined in skin components (epidermis, hair follicle, dermis, sebaceous glands) by dot blotting and northern blotting of extracted RNA, and has been observed in skin sections by tissue *in situ* hybridisation with labelled antisense riboprobes which can detect specific messenger RNA (mRNA) species (Fig. 2.2). Gene regulation and function of the encoded protein has also been studied by transient transfection of cultured cells with complete or modified genes (deletions, rearrangements or additions made to the original sequence and regulatory regions attached to reporter genes). Experiments with transgenic mice (the stable introduction of human genes, gene fragments or modified genes into mouse oocytes to produce genetically altered embryos) have also proved invaluable for studying gene expression and regulation in relation to embryonic development and tissue differentiation. Thus, these powerful molecular approaches have led to a greater understanding of the many structural proteins that come together to make up the different facets of a complex tissue such as the skin.

The purpose of this chapter is to give an overview of keratin gene expression in the skin, hair and nail, as well as looking briefly at other structural proteins involved in both epidermal-specific and hair-specific differentiation.

HISTORICAL PERSPECTIVES OF KERATIN

A multiplicity of terminology has developed within the keratin field over the last 40 years, and some of the most common terms are listed in Table 2.3. The

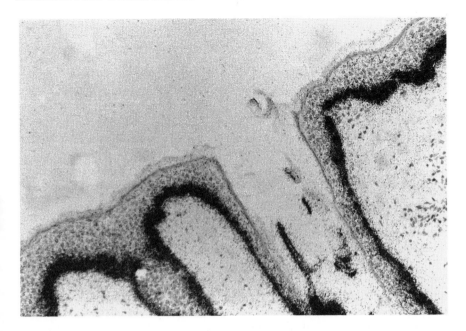

Fig. 2.2. *In situ* hybridisation on human skin sections with a riboprobe to human keratin 14. The mRNA encoding keratin 14 is clearly localised in the basal layer of the epidermis. Courtesy of Drs G. Parker and M.B. Hodgins, University of Glasgow, UK

Table 2.3. Keratin terminology

Kerat(o)	Greek word element for horn or horny tissues
Keratin	Insoluble proteinaceous substance (scleroprotein) of skin, hair, nail, wool, claw, hoof, horn, feather and scale
Soft keratins	Keratins of soft tissues (e.g. skin)
Hard keratins	Keratins of hard tissues (hair, nail, claw, etc.)
α-Keratins	Keratins with α-type X-ray diffraction pattern (e.g. wool, hair, skin). Protein in α-helical conformation
β-Keratins	Keratins with β-type X-ray diffraction pattern (e.g. scale and feather of birds and reptiles)
Low-sulphur keratins	Wool and hair microfibrillar IF keratins of low cysteine content (see Table 2.4)
High-sulphur keratins	Wool and hair matrix proteins of high cysteine content (also ultra-high-sulphur keratins; see Table 2.4)
Cytokeratins	Keratin IF proteins of epithelial cells as distinct from the specialised keratins of skin and hair
Epidermin	6 M urea extract of epidermis containing various keratins and other urea-soluble proteins
Prekeratin	Citric acid-soluble keratin complex from living epidermal cells. Precursor of the insoluble keratins of the horny layer

term *keratin* is derived from *keratos*, the Greek word for horn, and the outer surface of the skin (stratum corneum or cornified layer) is often called *the horny layer*. Thus, 'keratin' is often used in a general sense to describe the material substance of skin, hair, nail, horn, scale and feather, and very little was known about the protein components of this complex substance when these definitions were introduced. Keratins are sometimes referred to as *soft keratins* (those of the skin) and *hard keratins* (those of the hardened epithelial structures such as hair, wool, nail, claw, hoof, horn, feather and scale). In fact, examination of cattle horn shows that it is composed of a material that resembles matted hair, demonstrating a close relationship between materials that superficially appear quite different. As will become apparent, these soft and hard tissues are composed of similar and quite closely related structural proteins, which differ in their chemical properties and so produce materials of a different nature. Bird feathers and reptile scales are also composed of 'hard keratins' in the general sense, but this material is quite different in structure, both at the microscopic level and at the molecular level (for review see Gregg and Rogers, 1986). In fact some of the earliest work on keratins demonstrated that the X-ray diffraction pattern of bird feather is of the β-type (Astbury and Marwick, 1932) while that of skin and wool keratins is of the α-type (Pauling and Corey, 1953). This forms the basis of the historical definition of α-keratins (skin), indicating that the component proteins adopt an α-helical conformation and β-keratins (feather), which adopt a β-pleated sheet structure. It is also interesting to note that in birds and snakes both types of keratin are found in close proximity (α-keratins in skin epidermis and β-keratins in feathers and hard scales).

In the late 1970s, an important connection was made between two fields of research. It was found that when extracted keratins were reassembled *in vitro*, they formed filamentous structures that could be visualised in the electron microscope. These structures resembled the intermediate filaments (IF) that had been described by cell biologists and were often seen in the cytoplasm of epithelial cells. They were initially regarded by electron microscopists as disaggregation products of microtubules or myosin filaments. It is now known that most cells contain IF in their cytoplasm and that the epidermis, hair follicle and nail bed have capitalised on the keratin IF multigene family, in combination with other gene families of structural proteins, to build the tough, flexible, insoluble and relatively impenetrable structures (horny layer, hair and nail respectively) that provide protection against the harsh environment.

Historically, other terms have also been used in the general literature on materials that we commonly say are composed of keratin. For example, *epidermin* was used to describe a mixture of keratins and other proteins extracted from mammalian epidermis with 6 M urea. The protein complex, which is soluble in citric acid and can be purified from living epidermal cells or keratinocytes (cells that synthesise keratin), has been called *prekeratin*. This material was composed of several polypeptide chains and was described as the precursor of the insoluble disulphide cross-linked keratin found in the dead outer surface layers of the skin (the stratum corneum or horny layer composed of corneocytes). *Cytokeratin* is a term used by cell biologists and pathologists to describe the IF proteins found in the cytoplasm of epithelial cells and to distinguish them from the 'specialised keratins' of skin, wool, hair, hoof and horn. However, it is now known that all these different IF proteins belong to the same multigene family, and as they are all intracellular proteins the term cytokeratin would seem to be redundant. A further complication in terminology was also introduced from the Australian research on wool keratins, and is attributed to the sulphur content of these proteins (Table 2.4). Extracts of wool contained proteins of different amino acid composition and a classification based on the content of cysteine (a sulphur-containing amino acid) was introduced (low-sulphur keratins, high-sulphur keratins and ultra-high-sulphur keratins). This was further complicated by the finding that some structural proteins in wool had very little cysteine but were rich in glycine and tyrosine (called high-glycine–tyrosine proteins or HGTP; the term keratin is not generally used in this context). The low-sulphur wool keratins are now known to belong to the IF multigene family and the high (and ultra-high)-sulphur keratins are related to epidermal matrix proteins, a different gene family. Thus, for clarity, it has been suggested that the high (and ultra-high)-sulphur keratins of wool should be termed high (and ultra-high)-sulphur matrix proteins.

A few final points should be made regarding terminology. The cornea of the eye is epithelial in nature and structurally related to the epidermis, and the original Greek base word [kerat(o)] has given rise to medical terminology relevant to the cornea (*keratalgia, keratectasia, keratectomy, keratitis, keratocyte, keratoglobus, keratomalacia,* etc.) but not necessarily relevant to keratins. Also, two more areas of confusion sometimes arise especially when talking (as opposed to reading or writing) about keratins. Keratins should not be confused with *carotenes,* the plant pigments which are precursors of retinol (vitamin A). Nor should they be confused with *keratan* (normally referred to as keratan sulphate), a sulphated complex carbohydrate (glycosaminoglycan or GAG) which is a component of the proteoglycans found in the extracellular matrix of cartilage.

Table 2.4. Wool (hair) structural proteins ('keratins')

Protein type	Location	Amino acid content	Size range[a]
Low sulphur[b]	Microfibrils	1–3 mol% cysteine	38–53 kDa
High sulphur	Fibre matrix	20–30 mol% cysteine	11–26 kDa
Ultra-high sulphur	Matrix/cuticle	> 30 mol% cysteine	> 20 kDa
High Gly–Tyr	Matrix	20–40 mol% glycine	6–9 kDa
		12–20 mol% tyrosine	6–9 kDa

[a]Molecular mass (weight) range in kilodaltons (kDa).
[b]The low-sulphur proteins that form microfibrils of the hair (wool) shaft are keratin intermediate filament (IF) proteins. These hair-specific keratins have a higher cysteine content than other IF proteins (generally < 1 mol%). Data from Powell and Rogers (1986).

INTERMEDIATE FILAMENT PROTEINS

The abundant low-sulphur α-type keratins found in various epithelial cells of the skin and its appendages (epidermal keratinocytes, outer root sheath of the hair follicle, sebaceous gland duct, sweat gland duct, hair, wool, nail, claw, hoof and horn) are members of a large multigene family of closely related IF proteins (see Franke et al., 1982; Nagle, 1988; Steinert & Roop, 1988 for reviews). The IF proteins are major components of the cytoskeleton of most, if not all, eukaryotic cells and they display considerable structural and functional heterogeneity. About 40 individual IF proteins have been described to date, and the multigene family is much more complex than that of other cytoskeletal components: microfilaments are composed largely of α, β and γ-actin and microtubules are composed of α and β-tubulin. Cytoplasmic IF proteins are related to structural proteins that comprise the eukaryotic cell nuclear envelope (lamins A and C; see Krohne and Benavente, 1986, for a review), and it is generally accepted that both filament systems converge on the nuclear pore to provide structural integrity throughout the cell. IF proteins have also been tentatively identified in plant cells, yeasts and other simple eukaryotes, and preliminary information suggests that the structural proteins of cellular flagella (tektins), may also be members of the IF multigene family.

Cells of different embryonic origin have IF that are composed of different members of the IF family. The IF proteins were originally divided into five classes based on biochemical and immunological data (keratins, vimentin, desmin, glial fibrillary acidic protein and neurofilaments). However, in the light of more recent sequence data and information on gene structure, the original classification has been reorganised into five types (I–V) of IF protein (Table 2.5). Keratins are the most diverse and, unlike the other IF proteins, are obligate heteropolymers (filament formation requires at least one type I keratin and one type II keratin). To date, 16 human acidic (type I) keratin IF proteins have been described, ranging in size from 40 to 65 kDa and covering the acidic pH range

Table 2.5. Intermediate filament (IF) protein classification

Type	IF protein	Number	Size range	Tissue expression
I	Keratins (acidic)	≈16	40–65 kDa	Epithelia (keratinocytes)[a]
II	Keratins (basic)	≈13	50–70 kDa	Epithelia (keratinocytes)[a]
III	Peripherin	1	57 kDa	Peripheral nerves
	Vimentin	1	53 kDa	Mesenchymal (fibroblast)
	Desmin	1	52 kDa	Myogenic cells
	GFAP[b]	1	50 kDa	Astrocytes (glial cells)
IV	Neurofilaments	3	60–150 kDa	Neurones (CNS)
	α-Internexin	1	66 kDa	Neurones
V	Lamins (A, C)	≈4	60–70 kDa	Nuclear lamina (all cells)

[a]Keratins are expressed in epithelial cells as type I acidic–type II basic 'pairs'.
[b]Glial fibrillary acidic protein.

(p*I* 4.5–6). Only 13 human neutral–basic (type II) keratins have been characterised and they are somewhat larger (50–70 kDa) and more basic (p*I* 6.5–8.5) than type I keratins. Mesenchymal cells, such as dermal fibroblasts, express a single type III protein (vimentin) and myogenic cells express another type III protein (desmin). Astrocytes and glial cells express glial fibrillary acidic protein (GFAP; type III) while neuronal cells express peripherin (type III), one or more of the neurofilament triplet (NF-L, NF-M, NF-H) and α-internexin (type IV proteins). Lamins A and C, which form the nuclear lamina complex on the inner surface of the nuclear membrane of all eukaryotic cells, constitute type V IF proteins. Finally, another IF-related protein (nestin) has been identified in developmentally regulated stem cells (not found in adult cells) and tentatively placed in a separate class (type VI). While there appears to be considerable diversity among the members of the IF protein multigene family, they all make filamentous or mesh-like cellular structures based on a common theme: the α-helical nature of the central rod domain.

INTERMEDIATE FILAMENT STRUCTURE

The major structural characteristic of all IF proteins is the central α-helical rod domain, which is highly conserved both in size (310–315 amino acid residues for types I–IV and 355 residues for type V) and structure (Fig. 2.3). The characteristic feature is the quasi-heptad repeat $(a\text{-}b\text{-}c\text{-}d\text{-}e\text{-}f\text{-}g)_n$, where positions a and d are usually occupied by apolar amino acid residues and the other positions are occupied by polar or charged residues. This gives rise to an α-helical twist in the polypeptide chain favouring the formation of a coiled-coil

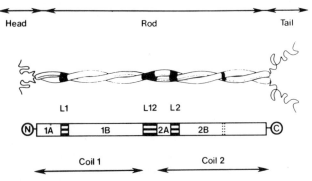

Fig. 2.3. A schematic diagram of the basic structure of an intermediate filament protein. The individual polypeptide chains or subunits have a central rod domain consisting of four α-helical regions (1A, 1B, 2A, 2B) separated by non-helical linkers (L1, L12, L2). The central domain is flanked by an amino terminal domain (head) and carboxy terminal domain (tail). The coiled-coil dimer shown is the result of hydrophobic interactions between the 'in-register' α-helical domains of the two component polypeptide chains. Courtesy of Prof. R. Nagle, University of Arizona, Tucson, USA

structure, and producing a characteristic surface pattern of charged and hydrophobic residues. The IF proteins have four such coiled-coil domains (1A, 1B, 2A and 2B) which are separated by short linker regions (L1, L12 and L2). Furthermore, in the 2B helical domain there is a conserved discontinuity in the regular pattern of the heptad repeat (Fig. 2.3). The central rod domain is about 47 nm long (each half [1A–L1–1B and 2A–L2–2B] is about 22 nm) and accounts for about 38 kDa in molecular weight terms. Thus the smallest keratin (K19), which is only 40 kDa, possesses a rod domain with only a minimal amount of amino (N) and carboxy (C) terminal sequences. It is these N- and C-terminal sequences that are largely responsible for the heterogeneity of IF proteins, both in terms of size (the termini account for 2–32 kDa) and composition (variable and unusual). While the sequence of the rod domains for IF proteins of the same type is highly conserved (60–75% homology), less conservation (30–40% homology) is observed between types, including type I and type II keratins. However, the terminal sequences (especially the C-terminus) are often unique and have highly specialised primary and secondary structures which differ not only between different types of IF protein but also between the different keratins.

Keratins are obligate heteropolymers, requiring more than one polypeptide chain or subunit to produce a filament, while desmin, vimentin and GFAP can all form homopolymeric filaments. The first step of IF protein polymerisation involves dimer formation (Fig. 2.4). This is a homodimer in the case of vimentin and other type III proteins, but the structure of keratin dimers is still a matter of some dispute (a heterodimer is favoured over two type-specific homodimers). Two dimers then condense to form an antiparallel staggered tetramer (Fig. 2.4) which in the case of keratins has two type II and two type I subunits. These aggregate with other tetrameric units to form an eight-chain unit and eventually a filament of 10–15 nm diameter. It is thought that the filaments form a lattice structure that has approximately 32 polypeptide chains in cross-section and shows axial repeats (by electron microscopy and X-ray diffraction) of 22 nm (half the length of the rod domain) and 47 nm (full length of central rod domain). The filaments themselves can be micrometres in length and form three-dimensional networks throughout the cell (see Fig. 2.1). They often aggregate together to form tonofilament bundles which run through the cellular cytoplasm and terminate at the desmosomal complexes that 'rivet' adjacent keratinocytes together (Fig. 2.5).

The bulk of the filament, as demonstrated by scanning transmission electron microscopy (STEM), is composed of the aligned rod domains which gives rise to the characteristic α-type X-ray diffraction pattern. However, the filaments appear 'fuzzy' at the surface and the density falls off at the periphery (cross-sectional analysis). This indicates that the N- and C-terminal sequences, which are quite extensive for the larger keratins and the neurofilaments, lie on the surface of the filament and protrude into the cytoplasm. In the case of

Keratin Heterodimer (Type II-Type I)

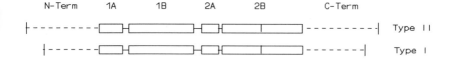

Half Staggered Anti-Parallel Tetramer

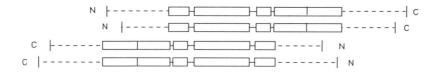

Possible Arrangement of Octameric Unit

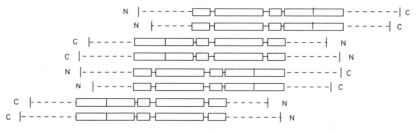

Fig. 2.4. A schematic diagram of IF protein subunits showing a keratin heterodimer, a half-staggered anti-parallel tetramer and the possible arrangement of an octameric unit. These are the favoured structural intermediates based on present knowledge. Vimentin and other type III IF proteins form 'in-register homodimers', but it is still possible that keratin IF proteins can form a heterotetramer composed of a type I homodimer and a type II homodimer

neurofilaments, protrusions have been seen in the electron microscope and they can form cross-bridges between filaments, as well as between neurofilaments and microtubules. Other evidence from studies of epidermal keratins also suggests that the termini are on the surface, as proteolytic modification and phosphorylation of intact filaments produces molecular alterations to the terminal sequences. As the IF proteins all differ in the nature of their terminal sequences, and these are accessible to the surrounding cellular environment, it appears that the function of individual IF proteins is dictated by the nature of these heterogeneous terminal ('surface') structures.

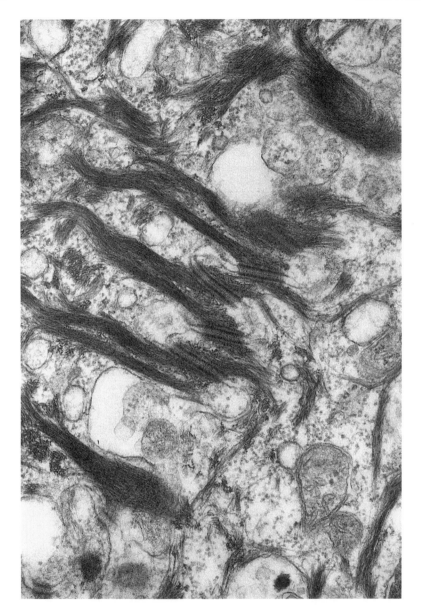

Fig. 2.5. Electron micrograph of keratin intermediate filaments. These often form large tonofilament bundles in suprabasal keratinocytes which terminate in desmosomal complexes at the plasma membrane of adjacent cells. Kindly provided by Dr W.E. Parish

INTERMEDIATE FILAMENT ASSOCIATED PROTEINS

A large number of accessory proteins are essential for the structure and function of both microfilaments (MF) and microtubules (MT). Both actin (the major structural protein of MF) and tubulin (the major structural protein of MT) are less diverse than IF proteins and are known to have many associated proteins. Actin, for example, has a plethora of binding proteins which confer many essential functions on the filaments themselves: they strengthen (tropomyosin), bundle (α-actinin, actinogelin, fascin, filamin, fimbrin, villin), fragment (brevin, depactin, gelsolin, severin, villin), slide along one another (myosin), move vesicles along (minimyosin), cap (α-actinin), attach to membranes (calspectin, spectrin, vinculin, talin), attach to extracellular matrix (connectin) and sequester monomers from the filament (profilin). Tubulin appears to have a smaller number of microtubule-associated proteins (ankyrin, dynein, kinesin, MAP-1, MAP-2 or tau proteins, nexin) which function to cross-link and attach microtubules to other filaments and cellular structures. The intermediate filament network also has a requirement for such accessory proteins and these have been termed IF-associated proteins (IFAPs).

Initially, it was thought that in contrast to the uniformity of actin and tubulin, IF proteins were so diverse that the variable termini of the molecules could perform all of the functions required. However, many cytoskeletal preparations that were free of actin and tubulin contained various co-purifying proteins. These could not be identified as being IF proteins present in minor quantities and were consistently present in cellular extracts. Meticulous isolation of a few of these proteins has shown that they are IFAPs which are generally present at levels much lower than the IF proteins themselves (1–10%). These IFAPs are responsible for the supramolecular organisation of IF networks and are proteins that can join filaments together, or anchor them to membranes and junctional complexes (e.g. desmosome, hemidesmosome). The matrix and envelope cross-linking proteins that are involved in epidermal differentiation (loricrin, filaggrin, involucrin) and hair differentiation (high-sulphur proteins, ultra-high-sulphur proteins, glycine–tyrosine-rich proteins and trichohyalin) can also be considered IFAPs that, like the keratin IF proteins, have been expressed to a high level in order to provide structural integrity to these specialised tissues. Paranemin and synemin are IFAPs that have been isolated from the erythrocyte cytoskeleton and muscle tissue, and these cross-link desmin and vimentin IF networks. Plectin and epinemin are ubiquitous IFAPs found at cellular anchoring sites (focal adhesions) and they bind filament systems together (IF and MT) as well as bind IF proteins to the plasma and nuclear membrane anchoring proteins. Spectrin, calspectin, ankyrin, lamin B and desmoplakin all serve as anchoring proteins but can also be considered as IF capping proteins. NAPA-73 and α-internexin are both associated with neurofilament IF proteins but their functions have not yet been defined (NAPA-73 is involved in neuronal development and α-internexin is homologous to the heat shock protein, HSP-70). Several other proteins have been described that are associated with the IF network but the results are currently too preliminary to report. This area of research is still in its infancy and more IFAPs must be awaiting discovery.

INTERMEDIATE FILAMENT GENES

The last 10 years have seen a tremendous increase in the understanding of intermediate filament structure and function, due to the application of molecular genetic techniques and advances in biochemistry and electron microscopy. While some protein sequences were available for wool keratins, a rapid increase in sequence information has allowed a detailed comparison of the diverse members of the IF multigene family. The first cDNA sequences were published in the early 1980s and the first IF gene sequence (vimentin) was completed at that time. It was followed by the desmin gene a year later and then by several keratin genes (K1, K6, K14, K16). Some IF genes were not cloned until the late 1980s and the gene sequences of the neurofilament triplet (NF-L, NF-M, NF-H), the lamins (A, C) and some of the hair-specific keratins have only been elucidated very recently. Several IF genes have not yet been cloned and fully characterised, and it is still debatable whether they have all been identified.

The IF genes of types I–III are remarkably conserved in structure and show common intron/exon boundaries. Type I keratin genes have eight exons (seven introns) while type II keratin genes and the type III genes (vimentin, desmin, GFAP) all have nine exons (eight introns). Two of the intron/exon boundaries in the 1B helix coding region and three boundaries in the 2B helix coding region are positionally conserved in all type I–III genes. The third boundary in the 1B helix region is conserved between type II and type III genes but different in type I genes. The type II keratins also have an intron/exon boundary in the 1B helix region and no boundaries have been found within the N-terminal coding sequences (refer to Fig. 2.6). However, type I–III genes all have a conserved intron/exon boundary in the first part of the C-terminal coding sequences and the type III genes have a second boundary in the middle of the C-terminal sequences. The neurofilament genes have a somewhat different structure and have only three introns: two in the 2B helix coding sequences (at different positions to type I–III genes) and the other in the C-terminal sequences (again at a unique location).

The different types of IF gene are spread throughout the genome and have been localised to separate chromosomes (Table 2.6). Desmin, vimentin and GFAP genes are all on different chromosomes (2, 10 and 17 respectively) and the neurofilament genes have been localised to two chromosomes (NF-L and NF-M on 8; NF-H on 22). However, several type I keratin genes show the same localisation and form two clusters: one on the short arm and the other on the

Table 2.6. Chromosomal localisation of human IF protein genes

IF type	IF genes	Chromosome
I	Keratins (K1, K4, K8)	12q[a]
II	Keratins (K10, K13, K14, K15, K16, K17, K19)	17 and q[b]
III	Desmin	2q
	Vimentin	10p
	GFAP	17
IV	Neurofilament (NF-L, NF-M)	8p
	Neurofilament (NF-H)	22q

[a]K18 is a type I keratin which has been mapped to the type II cluster on chromosome 12. However, *in situ* hybridisation data indicate that K18 resides on chromosome 17 and this point needs further clarification.
[b]Type I keratin genes have been traced to at least two different regions of chromosome 17. One cluster contains pseudogenes and more detailed investigation is required.

long arm of chromosome 17. The type II keratin genes that have been localised so far occur in a single cluster on the long arm of chromosome 12. There is confusion over the localisation of keratin 18 as this gene has been mapped to chromosome 12 by one group and to chromosome 17 by another, and its exact localisation awaits confirmation.

Present information suggests that IF genes occur as a single functional copy per haploid genome but there are reports for the keratins of the existence of pseudogenes (non-expressed genes either lacking introns, regulatory sequences or having in-frame stop codons that interrupt the encoded sequence). There are two similar clusters of type I keratin genes on chromosome 17 and one of these clusters contains pseudogenes. Thus, it is still not clear exactly how many IF genes exist and, while there are at least 40 (one for each encoded IF protein), the existence of multiple copies cannot be ruled out at present. There have also been reports of alternate splicing for the vimentin gene and at least two mRNA transcripts have been identified. These transcripts only differ in the non-coding portions of the mRNA and appear to produce identical proteins, the expression of which can be regulated differently at the level of vimentin mRNA in different cells. Exactly how widespread alternate splicing is as a regulatory mechanism amongst the IF genes is not yet known.

The several theories concerning the evolution of IF genes are constantly being modified to accommodate new information. It is generally accepted that an ancestral gene existed earlier than 1000 million years ago. This gene probably had few, if any, introns and may be closely related to the IF lamin genes which arose in early eukaryotes at about this time. Thus, divergence of a single IF progenitor gene into a cytoplasmic and a nuclear counterpart was probably the first event. The neurofilament genes probably diverged from the cytoplasmic ancestral gene initially, as they have the simplest intron/exon structure of the cytoplasmic IF genes. The type I–III genes must have diverged later in evolutionary history and formed three distinct evolutionary conserved groups (types I, II and III). These theories have been based on computer predictions of the relatedness of helical rod domain sequences (Blumenberg,

1989) and do not explain the occurrence of the hypervariable N- and C-terminal domains of the IF proteins. To date, the information on gene structure, sequence and expression has been of little help in explaining the recruitment of the specialised end domains onto the various type-specific rod domains. The evolution of these genes will remain an intriguing question for some time to come and may provide valuable information regarding the evolutionary development of organisms that have a complex array of differentiated cell types from more simple life forms.

KERATIN EXPRESSION IN DIVERSE EPITHELIA

The epithelial cell-specific keratins are the most diverse class of IF proteins, and 30 individual human keratins, ranging from 40 to 70 kDa in size, have so far been described (Moll et al., 1982; Heid et al., 1988). Keratins are divided into two distinct groups: the smaller acidic type I keratins and the larger basic–neutral type II keratins. These are all encoded by different genes and in some instances more than one gene has been identified for a particular keratin IF protein. However, in these circumstances, the additional genes have all been designated pseudogenes of one sort or another, and are not expressed in epithelial tissues. Not all keratins are expressed by individual types of epithelial cell (Table 2.7) and, typically, two to ten different keratins are expressed per cell type in various 'functional' combinations. Thus, keratins are not only epithelial specific but also show further functional diversity (different keratins

Table 2.7. Human keratin IF proteins

Tissue expression[a]	Type II basic (size)[b]	Type I acidic (size)
Epidermis, upper duct (PSU)	K1, K2 (68, 65 kDa)	K9,[c] K10[d] (65, 57 kDa)
Cornea (eye)	K3 (64 kDa)	K12 (55 kDa)
Oesophagus, internal organs	K4 (59 kDa)[e]	K13, K20 (54, 46 kDa)
Epidermis, hair follicle (ORS)	K5 (60 kDa)	K14, K15 (51, 50 kDa)
Epidermis,[f] hair follicle (ORS)	K6 (58 kDa)	K16, K17 (49, 49 kDa)
Sweat gland, sebaceous gland	K7 (55 kDa)	K19 (40 kDa)[g]
Simple epithelia (e.g. liver, kidney)	K8 (54 kDa)	K18 (44 kDa)
Hair shaft and nail plate	HaKb1–4 (58–64 kDa)[h]	HaKa1–4 (42–46 kDa)[h]

[a]Keratins are heteropolymers and expressed in type I–type II pairs (e.g. K1–K10).
[b]Size of keratin IF proteins as determined by SDS–polyacrylamide gel electrophoresis.
[c]K9 is abundant in palmar and plantar epidermis but a minor component elsewhere.
[d]Another keratin (K11) similar in size to K10 has been described but not yet cloned.
[e]A 59 kDa keratin (not necessarily K4) has been found in palmar/plantar epidermis.
[f]K6 and K16 are constitutively expressed in the hair follicle and sebaceous gland duct but are only expressed in epidermis that is hyperproliferating.
[g]K19 is present in minor amounts at several locations including epidermal basal cells and the presumptive stem cell population of the hair follicle.
[h]Two hair-related keratins (Hbx, Hax) have been described and recently cloned.

are expressed in different epithelia), making the developmental regulation of these genes extremely interesting.

The largest keratins (K1, K2, K9, K10) are expressed in the differentiating cells of interfollicular epidermis (Table 2.7). However, K2 and K9 are generally minor components except in palmar/plantar epidermis where K9 and a basic 59 kDa keratin are major components of the filament system. K1 and K10 are also expressed in the upper portion of the pilosebaceous duct that is continuous with the epidermis and in the keratinising epithelium of the anal canal. In the mouse, K1 and K10 are also expressed in the forestomach, which in this species is a keratinising stratified epithelium like the epidermis.

The stratified epithelium of the cornea expresses K3 and K12 and these two keratins appear to be specific for this type of differentiation. The oesophagus, various internal organs, tongue, epiglottis and apocrine glands of the axilla express K4 and K13 in the differentiated cells. Recently, a smaller type I keratin (K20) has also been found in this type of epithelium. Most stratified epithelia (such as the oesophagus, cornea, epidermis and hair follicle) express K5 and K14 in the lower basal cells and in early differentiated cells. However, as differentiation proceeds in these epithelia, the filament network that is initially composed of K5 and K14 is changed by a high level of expression of the differentiation-specific keratins characteristic of the particular epithelia.

The outer root sheath cells of the hair follicle and cells of the sebaceous gland duct also express K5 and K14 but in addition constitutively express K6 and K16. These keratins are also constitutively expressed in palmar/plantar epidermis but are not found under normal circumstances in interfollicular epidermis, where their presence is an indication of hyperproliferation. Thus, K6 and K16 are expressed in response to any wounding or perturbation of the epidermis. K15 has been described as a minor component of the epidermis and hair follicle but only seems to be abundant in the epithelia of the eccrine sweat gland, epiglottis and trachea. K17 expression has been identified in the hair follicle, mammary gland duct and tracheal epithelium but as this keratin co-localises with K16 on most two-dimensional gel systems used for this type of analysis, and few monospecific antisera are available, the precise expression of K17 has not been completely documented.

Some stratified epithelia also express K7 and K19, and these keratins have been found in both apocrine and eccrine sweat glands, mammary gland ducts and tracheal epithelium. K19 has also been identified as a minor keratin in the epidermis and hair follicle, where it localises specifically to the germinative compartments where stem cells arise. The transitional epithelia of the bladder and gallbladder express K7 and K19 in addition to the keratins characteristic of simple epithelia (K8, K18). The simple mucosal epithelium of the small intestine and colon, and the simple epithelia of other internal organs such as the liver and kidney, have the simplest keratin expression, consisting only of K8 and K18, although some K19 expression is often observed.

Finally, it has become apparent that the microfibrillar keratins of wool, hair and nail are a specialised subgroup of the IF keratins. These proteins were identified in wool extracts prior to the established nomenclature for human epithelial keratins (Moll *et al.*, 1982), when human hair and nail keratins had not been adequately characterised. This has given rise to an anomaly in the simple classification of keratins (K1–K19) introduced in 1982 to replace diverse molecular weight assignations, and the hair-specific keratins have been given a different nomenclature (HaKb1–4 and HaKa1–4). Furthermore, another epithelial keratin has since been identified in the epithelial cells of some internal organs (K20) and two other keratins have been identified in the nail plate and dorsal mucosa of the tongue (Hbx and Hax). These two keratins are related to, but distinct from, hair-specific keratins and have recently been found at high levels in the parakeratotic scales of mouse tail epidermis (Tobiasch *et al.*, 1992). Finally, Heid and co-workers (1988) found, surprisingly, that hair-specific keratins (including Hbx and Hax) were present in the epithelium of the thymus together with keratins normally expressed by the epithelial cells of internal organs. Exactly why these 'hard' keratins are required at this location can only be a matter of speculation. This is only a brief summary of the data available on keratin expression in various epithelia but it clearly demonstrates the considerable diversity and functional complexity of this multigene family of keratin IF proteins.

KERATIN SEQUENCE HOMOLOGY AND DIVERSITY

Most of the amino acid sequences available for keratin IF proteins have been deduced using the genetic code from sequence information determined at the DNA level. Keratins have been particularly difficult to handle in respect to direct protein purification and sequencing, but the protein sequence data that have been determined directly have agreed with the DNA-derived sequence. Classification of keratins into type I acidic and type II basic groups, originally done on the basis of biochemical and immunological data, has been confirmed by the more recent sequence data. The helical regions of different type II keratins are highly homologous (Table 2.8) and a level of 67–87% sequence identity can be obtained at the amino acid level for 2B helical sequences. In general, over the whole helical region (including the linkers) homology in excess of 60% is obtained when comparing different type II keratins. This is also true of type I keratins (Table 2.8), although the percentage homology in the 2B helical region is somewhat more variable (47–95%). However, a particularly high level of homology exists between some human type I keratins (K14–K16, 92%; K14–K17, 93%; K16–K17, 95%) in the 2B helical region, while lower homology is obtained for K18 and K19 (47%). Sequence homology between type I and type II keratins is lower and typical values for the 2B helix are in the range 31–42%. This level of homology is also generally found amongst all of the IF proteins especially in the 2B helix, which is particularly well conserved.

In contrast, the N- and C-terminal regions of the different keratin IF proteins are quite unique and are thought to confer specific functions on the individual keratin pairs that are expressed in different epithelia. This can be appreciated by comparing the C-terminal sequences of various human keratins (Table 2.9). While certain trends can be identified, these sequences are quite distinct for a particular keratin and it is even hard to find reasonable homology between the co-expressed keratin pairs (e.g. K1–K10, K4–K13, K5–K14, K6–K16, K8–K18). Not only do the sequences themselves vary, but so does the length of the terminal sequence, as given in Table 2.9 by the number of residues beyond the highly conserved and characteristic 2B helix sequence (TYRxLLEGEE). These differences in the C-terminal sequences, as well as those in the N-terminal sequences (not shown), are not only responsible for the size and charge heterogeneity by which the individual keratins have been classified, but also for the functional heterogeneity that is a consequence of the expression of these different protein sequences in epithelia with diverse biological capabilities. This can easily be seen by making a few comparisons of the sequence data and looking at the properties in general biochemical terms. For instance, both K1 and K10 have termini that are rich in glycine. Once removed by proteolytic cleavage, these termini exist as 15 kDa polypeptides that cannot be further degraded and are totally insoluble in an aqueous environment – properties that are ideally suited to existence on the skin surface. K6 and K16 termini seem to be particularly rich in serine, which is a major acceptor of phosphate in biological phosphorylation reactions and is probably important for regulating the function of these particular keratins. Finally, the hair-specific keratins contain the largest number of terminal cysteines amongst the IF proteins. While they are classified as low-sulphur keratins in terms of wool and hair proteins (see Table 2.4), these keratins are ideally adapted to forming hard structures by extensive disulphide bridging with the abundant high-sulphur matrix proteins found in the hair and nail. As more information about the biological nature of these terminal sequences becomes available, their cellular function will become less of a mystery, and may help to explain the bewildering diversity of keratin IF proteins expressed by epithelial cells.

KERATIN GENE STRUCTURE, LOCALISATION AND LINKAGE

Keratin gene structure is generally conserved in a type-specific manner, in that type II keratins have nine exons and eight introns while type I keratins have eight exons and seven introns. Furthermore, the location at which these introns interrupt the coding sequence is highly conserved (Fig. 2.6). However, there are exceptions to this general rule and at least three type I keratin genes are divergent in this respect. Both K18 and HaKa1 (a hair-specific keratin gene) do not have an intron in the C-terminal domain, yet the location of the other six

38

Table 2.8. Amino acid sequence[a] homology in the 2B α-helical region of human keratins

Keratin	Sequence	Homology[b]
Type II		
K1	QGENALKDAKNKLNDMEDALQQAKEDLARLLCDYHELMNTKLALDLEIATYRTLLEGEES	73%
	** ***** ** ****** ***** ** **** ****** ******	
K3	HGEMALKDANAKLQELQAALQQAKDDLARLLRDYQELMNVKLALDVEIATYRKLLEGEEY	78%
	** ***** * ****** ** *** ** ***** ************	
K4	RGENALKDAHSKRVELEAALQQAKEELARMLREYQELMSVKLALDIEIATYRKLLEGEEY	75%
	** ***** ** ** ** ** * * **********	
K5	RGELALKDARNKLAELEEALQKAKQDMARLLREYQELMNTKLALDVEIATYRKLLEGEEC	87%
	***** ****** ** ***** ** **** ******* ***********	
K6	RGEMALKDAKNKLEGLEDEALQKAKQDLARLLKEYQELMNVKLALDVEIATYRKLLEGEEC	77%
	** **** ** ** *** ***** ** ** ***** ****** ********	
K7	CGELALKDARAKQEELEAALQRAKQDMARQLREYQELMSVKLALDIEIATYRKLLEGEES	82%
	** *** ** ** ***** ****** ** ** ***************	
K8	RGEMAVKDAQAKLARLEAALRNAKQDMARQLREYQELMNVKLALDVEIATYRKLLEGEES	67%
	** * ** ** ** *** ** ***** ** ** ******	
Hb2	QGEAALSDRRCKLAELEGALQKAKQDMASLIREYQEVMNSKLGLDIEIATYRRLLEGEEQ	
Type I		
K10	RYCVQLSQIQAQISALEEQLQEIRAETECQNTEYQQLTDIKIRLENEIQTYRSLLEGEGS	63%
	** **** * ** *** ** **** ** *********	
K13	RYALQLQQIQGLISSIEAQLSELRSEMECQNQEYKMLLDIKTRLEQEIATYRSLLEGQDA	73%
	** **** * * *** ** ** ******* *** *********** **	
K14	RYCMQLAQIQEMIGSVEEQLAQLRCEMEQQNQEYKILLDVKTRLEQEIATYRRLLEGEDA	75%
	** **** ** ** ******* ****** *** *********** **	
K15	RYATQLQQIQGLIGGLEAQLSELRCEMEAQNQEYKMLLDIKTRLEQEIATYRSLLEGQDA	75%
	** **** ** *** ***** *** ******* *** ********** **	
K16	RYCMQLSQIQGLIGSVEEQLAQLRCEMEQQSQEYQILLDVKTRLEQEIATYRRLLEGEDA	95%
	** **************** ****** *** *********************	
K17	RYCVQLSQIQGLIGSVEEQLAQLRCEMEQQNQEYKILLDVKTRLEQEIATYRRLLEGEDA	50%
	** * ** *** ** *** ** *** ** *********** **	
K18	RYALQMEQLNGILLHLESELAQTRAEGQRQAQEYEALLNIKVKLEAEIATYRRLLEDGED	47%
	* * ** ** ** ** *** ** *** ********* **	
K19	RFGAQLAHIQALYSGIEAQLADVRADSERQNQEYQRLMDIKSRLEQEIATYRSLLEGQED	65%
	* * ** ** ** *********	
Ha1[3]	..............LERQNQEYQVLLDVRARLECEINTYRSLLESEDC	

[a] Amino acid sequences shown in single-letter code (e.g. R = arginine; G = glycine) and amino acid residue identity is shown (*) for adjacent keratin sequences.
[b] Sequence homologies (% identity) given for adjacent keratins (e.g. K1–K3 = 73%). About 35% homology is observed for the 2B helical regions of type II and type I keratins.
[c] Sequence of this human hair-specific keratin is still incomplete.

Table 2.9. Carboxy-terminal amino acid sequences[a] of human keratins

Keratin		C-term[b]
Type II		
K1	GGGGGGSSGGRGSGGGSGGSSGGSGGRGSSSGGVKSSGGSSVRFVSTSYSGVTR–	153 AA[b]
K3	GIGCGFGGGSGFSGCSGGSGFGSISGARYGVSGGGFSSASNRGGSIKFSQSSQSSQRYSR–	118 AA
K4	TGGISGCGLGSGSGFGLSSGFGSGSGSGFGFGSVSGSSSSKIISTTTLNKRR–	72 AA
K5	VGLGGGLSVGGSGFSASSRGLGVGFGSGGGSSSVKFVSTTSSSRKSFKS–	111 AA
K6	YSYGSGLGVGGGFSSSSGRAIGGGLSSVGGGSTIKYTTTSSSSRKSYKH–	90 AA
K7	SSSGGGIGLTLGGTMGSNALSFSSSAGPGLLKAYSIRTASASRRSARD–	68 AA
K8	GGLTSSYGTPGFNYSLSPGSFSRTSSKPVVVKIETRDGKLVSESSDVLSK–	71 AA
Hb2[c]	GAVNVCVSSSRGVVCGDLCVSGSRPVTGSVCSAPCNGNVAVSTDLCAPCAKLNTTC–	63 AA
Type I		
K10	SGGGGGGYGGGSSGGGSSSGGGYGGGSSSGGGYGGGSSSGGHKSSSSGSVGESSSKGPRY–	109 AA[b]
K13	KMIGFPSSAGSVSPRSTSVTTTSSASVTTTSNASGRRTSDVRRP*	44 AA
K14	HRQIRTKVMDVHDGKVVSTHEQVLRTKN*	28 AA
K15	KMAGIGIREASSGGGSSSNFHINVEESVDGQVVSSHKREI*	41 AA
K16	HLSSQQASGQSYSSREVFTSSSSSAVRPGPSSEQSSSSFSQGQSS*	46 AA
K17	HLTQYKKEPVTTRQVRTIVEEVQDGKVISSREQVHQTTR–	39 AA
K18	FNLGDALDSSNSMQTIQKTTTRRIVDGKVVSETNDTKVLRH–	41 AA
K19	HYNNLSASKVL–	11 AA
Ha1[c]	KLPSNPCATTNACSKPIGPCLSNPCTSCVPPAPCTPCAPRPRCGPCNSFVR–	51 AA

[a] Amino acid sequences shown in single letter code (e.g. R = arginine).
[b] Number of amino acid residues in carboxy terminus (beyond 2B Helix).
[c] Hair-specific keratins have a large number of cysteine residues (**C**).

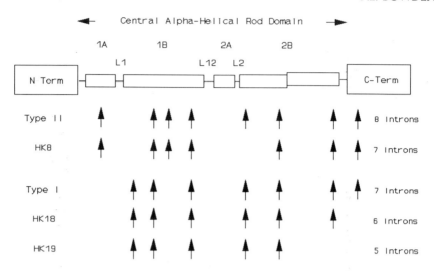

Fig. 2.6. A schematic diagram of IF protein structure showing the positions along the length of the protein where introns interrupt the coding sequence. While the positioning of intron–exon boundaries is highly conserved in both type II and type I keratin genes, the number of introns has been found to vary and the known exceptions are shown

introns is highly conserved (Fig. 2.6). Furthermore, K19 lacks both the intron in the C-terminal domain and the intron at the end of the 2B helix. Again the other five introns in the K19 gene are positionally conserved. Type II keratin genes show less variability but the K8 gene is exceptional. Intron V, located at the beginning of the 2B helix, is missing in the K8 gene, which therefore has only seven introns in total. As more genes are isolated and sequenced, perhaps a definite pattern of the location of intron/exon boundaries will emerge and throw more light on the evolution of these genes.

Keratin genes are not scattered widely throughout the genome but exist in two defined clusters that are type specific (Fig. 2.7; Table 2.6). The type II keratin gene cluster is located on the long arm of chromosome 12 (12q11–13), while there appear to be two clusters of type I keratin genes – one on the short arm and one on the long arm of chromosome 17 (17p12 and 17q11.2). Several groups have demonstrated that keratin genes are linked together in these clusters and there is little evidence for linkage of type I and type II genes. There may be one exception to the type-specific clustering rule, as human K18 (type I keratin) has been mapped to chromosome 12 (type II locus). However, another group have localised the K18 gene to the type I cluster on chromosome 17 by *in situ* hybridisation and this matter has yet to be resolved. A systematic approach to mapping the chromosomal localisation of all keratin genes has not yet been attempted, but all the available evidence points to these two separate loci, suggesting that the genes evolved from a pair of progenitor genes by duplication and sequence diversification.

Several pseudogenes, both processed and mutated whole genes, have been

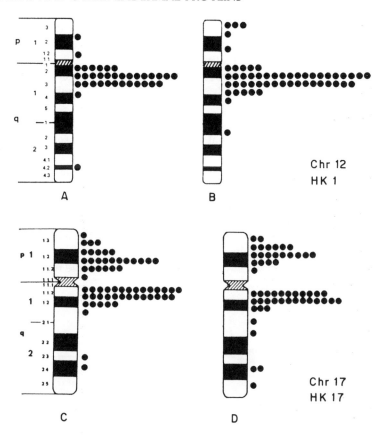

Fig. 2.7. A schematic diagram of chromosomal *in situ* hybridisation showing the localisation of a type II human keratin gene (HK1) to chromosome 12 (A: Pst 800 bp probe to the 3' non-coding region of a type II gene upstream of HK1; B: Bam HI-Pst I 2100 bp probe to the 3' non-coding region of HK1) and a type I human keratin gene (HK17) to chromosome 17 (C: PCR-generated 236 bp probe to the C-terminal and 3' non-coding sequences of HK17; D: Bam HI 1400 bp cDNA probe covering coding and 3' non-coding sequences of HK17). The dots represent a semi-quantitative grain count of over 70 metaphase chromosome spreads. Work done in collaboration with Dr N. Popescu, National Institutes of Health, USA (see Popescu *et al.*, 1989)

described to date but these are mostly type I keratins. One human K14 pseudogene recently characterised has three frameshift mutations in coding sequences (one duplication, one deletion and one insertion), two altered intron/extron boundaries and an altered polyadenylation signal. Two pseudogenes have been identified for human K17 which have in-frame stops in the coding sequence and regions that are duplicated. A processed pseudogene (no introns) has been found for human K19 and this gene is 82% homologous to the coding sequence of the transcribed normal gene. Also, a complete and apparently functional copy of the human K16 gene has been characterised but is not expressed. There is preliminary evidence that one of the two type I gene clusters on chromosome 17 is composed entirely of pseudogenes, and this may be the reason that type I keratin pseudogenes appear more prevalent. However, a mouse K8 (type II) processed pseudogene has been reported, and several human K8 pseudogenes have been identified by polymerase chain reaction (PCR).

The overall size of the keratin gene clusters is presently unknown. However, the available evidence suggests that the genes are linked closely together, as between two and four genes can be isolated on single lambda or cosmid clones (20–40 kb of DNA). In general, type I genes are closer together and individual cosmid clones with inserts of 35–40 kb contain two or three keratin genes spaced by about 5–7 kb (Fig. 2.8). Type II keratin genes are more spread out, as only one or two genes are obtained on single cosmid clones, and these are spaced by 10–15 kb (Fig. 2.8). Systematic chromosome walking or the isolation of large fragments of genomic DNA in yeast artificial chromosomes (YACs) should allow complete characterisation of these genetic loci over the next few years.

A)   Type II Keratin Gene Cluster (Chr 12)

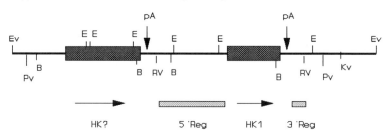

B)   Type I Keratin Gene Cluster (Chr 17)

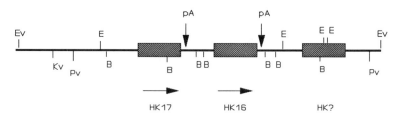

Fig. 2.8. A schematic diagram of keratin gene structure showing the location of regulatory sequences both upstream (5'Reg) and downstream (3'Reg) of the gene and of the polyadenylation signals (pA). Keratin genes are linked together and an example of each type of cluster is shown (A: type II genes on chromosome 12; B: type I genes on chromosome 17). These linked genes were identified on individual human cosmid clones. The direction of transcription (→) and several restriction enzyme sites (E = Eco RI, B = Bam HI, RV = Eco RV, K = Kpn I, P = Pst I; Ev, Kv, Pv designate RE sites in cosmid vector) are labelled

KERATIN GENE REGULATION

Studies of keratin gene regulation are still in their infancy, but now that several complete genes have been isolated and characterised the understanding of their regulation is a major goal. Sequence comparison of the upstream regions (5' non-coding) of several keratin genes, including co-expressed pairs, has yielded very little in terms of characterising the elements responsible for tissue-specific and differentiation-specific regulation. Comparison of the upstream regulatory regions of the genes that encode human K5 and K14 (a co-expressed pair) showed that no particular regions are conserved with respect to regulatory elements, indicating that common sequence motifs are not necessary for coordinate expression of keratin pairs. More progress has been made by functional studies of prospective regulatory regions upstream of the genes (5' non-coding), within the introns, and downstream (3' non-coding). Such studies involve the transient transfection of constructs containing the prospective regulatory region coupled to a reporter gene (chloramphenicol acetyltransferase, CAT; β-galactosidase; luciferase) into suitable cells (3T3 fibroblasts or various epithelial cells; COS, PtK2, MDBK, keratinocytes). The precise regulatory element can then be identified by progressive deletion of the surrounding DNA and by subjecting a series of modified constructs to functional assay (e.g. CAT assay). Gel retardation or band-shift assays can also be performed, in addition to DNA protection assays, to confirm the existence of a functional regulatory element. Finally, transgenic mice have proved particularly useful for the study of gene regulation as precise details of the developmental-specific, tissue-specific and differentiation-specific expression can be examined as the mice develop.

Recent experiments have determined that the human K1 gene has an epidermal-specific promoter upstream of the start of transcription (within 1.5 kb), a basal cell-specific silencer distal to the start of transcription (between − 9 kb and − 3 kb) and a calcium-responsive element at the 3' end of the gene. In addition, sequencing of the region upstream of the HK1 gene has identified several known eukaryotic gene regulatory elements (Sp1, Sph, PEA3, octamer) at distances up to 10 kb from the start of transcription. An 18 kb fragment of DNA (Eco RV), containing the complete human K1 gene, 3 kb of downstream sequence and 9 kb of upstream sequence, has all the regulatory elements necessary for specific and complete regulation of this gene in transgenic mice. A similar situation exists for the human K19 gene, which requires about 1 kb of downstream sequence and 8.6 kb of upstream sequence in addition to the complete gene for normal expression.

The mouse endo A gene (equivalent to human K8) has six direct repeats of the PEA3 motif (polyoma virus α-enhancer core) about 1 kb downstream of the gene which forms a functional promoter. The human K18 gene has a putative AP-1 site and three Sp-1 sites in the large first intron (2534 bp) which can be activated by two proto-oncogene DNA binding proteins (c-*fos* and c-*jun*). This gene has also been put into transgenic mice and has been shown to undergo normal regulation with 2.5 kb upstream flanking DNA and 3.5 kb downstream. Five human K18 genes have been described but only one is actively transcribed, demonstrating the importance of various negative elements (silencers) and DNA binding proteins for normal keratin gene expression. Furthermore in human fibroblasts and myoblasts, analysis of K18 genes has shown that the 5' flanking DNA is heavily methylated, which could be the mechanism by which keratin genes are permanently switched off in non-epithelial cells during embryonic development.

The human K7 gene is regulated differentially by retinoids, glucocorticoids and oestradiol in different epithelial cells, and this is due to the presence of various upstream elements that can bind retinoic acid receptors (RAR) and steroid hormone receptors. Evidence has been found for the presence of RAR and T3R (triiodothyronine receptor) responsive elements upstream of several keratin genes (e.g. K5, K6, K10 and K14). The human K14 gene is normally regulated in transgenic mice in the presence of 2.5 kb upstream flanking and 0.7 downstream sequence. A strong promoter region exists 300 bp up from the start of transcription of the K14 gene, but other elements further upstream are also needed. Smaller amounts of upstream flanking are sufficient for the normal regulation of K5 and K6 (1.2 kb) but this is not enough information to determine epidermal specificity for K10. Thus, it can be seen that the different keratin genes require different amounts of flanking DNA to invoke precise expression.

Various transcription factor binding motifs have also been found upstream of keratin genes as well as in introns. AP-2 sites have been found in the 5' flanking DNA of the K5 and K14 genes as well as in intron 2 of the K18 gene. Keratinocytes contain a transcription factor (called KER 1) and recent evidence suggests that this is identical to the AP-2 factor (Leask et al., 1991). However, while the AP-2 site is necessary for the transcription of K14, it is not sufficient to determine epidermal specificity for the expression of this gene. Another element (AARCCAA) that has been located upstream of some epidermal keratin genes is thought to confer epidermal specific expression, but this is distal to the start of transcription and no binding protein has been identified yet. Many sequence motifs and regulatory factors are known to influence the transcription of eukaryotic genes (Johnson and McKnight, 1989) and the keratin genes are no exception in this respect. These studies are still in their infancy, but it can be appreciated from this brief examination that keratin gene regulation is highly complex, requires up to 10 kb upstream flanking DNA, 3 kb downstream and functional introns. A totally functional and properly regulated transcription unit is therefore about 10–20 kb depending on the keratin gene involved. Much more research is required in this area and it will probably be some years before the precise developmental-specific and tissue-specific regulation of keratin genes is clearly defined.

KERATINS AND EPIDERMAL DIFFERENTIATION

The correct regulation of keratin gene expression and the formation of a functional keratin IF network are essential for normal epidermal differentiation. The epidermis of all mammals is a stratified squamous epithelium that undergoes a complex series of morphological and biochemical changes during the process of terminal differentiation (keratinisation). This culminates in the formation of the horny layer, which provides a durable, pliable and effective barrier of tightly packed dead cells (modified keratinocytes called corneocytes). In a total extract of detergent-soluble proteins (under reducing conditions) from human or mouse epidermis, 25–30% of the protein is made up of keratin IF. Three other types of structural protein are also found as major components of mammalian epidermis: filaggrin or histidine-rich protein (from keratohyalin granules), loricrin or cysteine-rich protein (also from keratohyalin granules) and involucrin (an envelope protein found in primates). More are probably awaiting discovery.

In addition to the proteins that make the filament-amorphous matrix of the epidermal cells, adjacent keratinocytes are held together by the desmosomal complex. The proteins of the desmosomes have also been characterised biochemically and some have recently been cloned and sequenced. Several plaque proteins have been identified (desmoplakin I, 250 kDa; desmoplakin II, 220 kDa; desmoplakin III or plakoglobin, 83 kDa; desmoplakin IV, 70 kDa; desmocalmin, 240 kDa) and other glycoproteins involved in transmembrane portions form the 'glue' in the extracellular space (desmogleins and desmocollins). Several of these components are the same in desmosomes and hemidesmosomes, but the latter have some unique structural components (bullous pemphigoid antigen, 230 kDa, and two other proteins of 180 kDa and 125 kDa). The cloning and sequencing data available for desmoplakins I and II have confirmed that these are related to the cadherin multigene family.

Four major constitutive keratins are expressed by human interfollicular epidermis (K1, K5, K10, K14), two more are expressed in hyperproliferative states (K6, K16) and two others are found in major amounts only in palmar/plantar skin (K9 and a 59 kDa basic keratin which migrates between K5 and K6 on gels). Minor amounts of K13, K15 and K19 have also been described in human epidermis. However, considering the major epidermal keratins only, expression alters during terminal differentiation. The basal cells of the epidermal proliferative compartment have a filament system that is not extensive and is composed largely of K5 and K14 (Fig. 2.9b). As cells become committed to terminal differentiation, they switch on two other keratin genes: K1 and K10. Evidence suggests that K1 expression precedes that of K10 and that once cells express these suprabasal keratins they must leave the basal layer. Biochemical, immunological and *in situ* hybridisation data show that K5 and K14 are progressively down-regulated and that the filament system in the

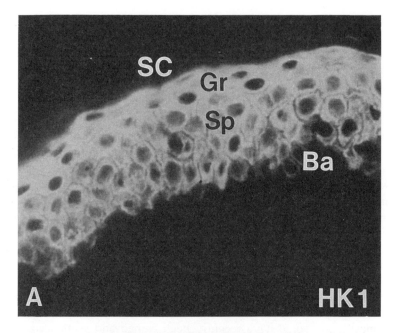

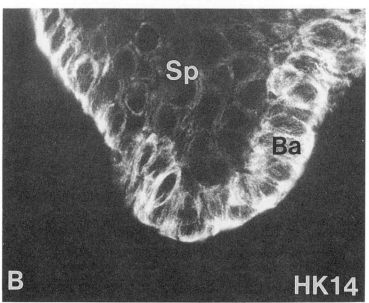

Fig. 2.9. Immunohistochemistry of human skin with specific antibodies to human keratins. (A) Expression of human keratin 1 (HK1) in suprabasal epidermal cells. Fluorescence staining of the cytoplasm of spinous (Sp) and granular (Gr) cells clearly visible. (B) Expression of human keratin 14 (HK14) in epidermal basal (Ba) cells. (Work done in collaboration with Professor Fusenig, Heidelberg, Germany (A) and data kindly provided by Prof. I.M. Leigh, London Hospital Medical College, UK(B).)

upper suprabasal cells not only increases in density but also changes in composition, as more K1–K10 appears. When the cells reach the upper granular layer, the filament system is composed almost entirely of K1 and K10 (Fig. 2.9a). These filaments are then proteolytically modified, becoming smaller and more acidic as the organelles are removed and the dead corneocytes are formed (Bowden *et al.*, 1987; Fig. 2.10).

The envelope protein involucrin (95 kDa) is expressed in upper spinous cells and is cross-linked to the plasma membrane by epidermal transglutaminases

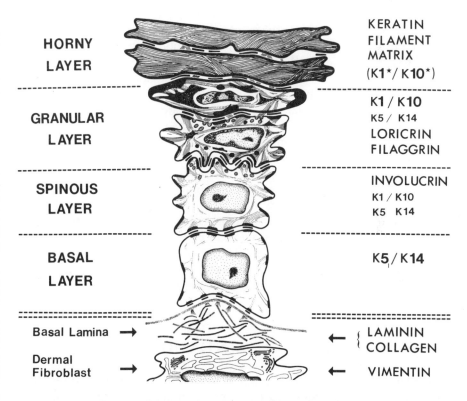

Fig. 2.10. A schematic diagram of epidermal differentiation showing the changes in keratinocyte morphology as differentiation proceeds and linking this to known alterations in the gene expression of the major structural proteins involved. Basal cells mainly express keratins K5 and K14, but when the cells are committed to terminal differentiation and destined to leave the basal layer, K1 and K10 expression is induced. The filaments of the spinous cells are composed of all four keratins but granular cells show mainly K1 and K10. The filaments in the horny layer are composed entirely of proteolytically modified keratins derived from K1 and K10. Involucrin expression occurs in the spinous layer but transglutaminase cross-linking to the plasma membrane does not occur until the upper granular layer. Filaggrin and loricrin expression occurs later in the granular layer and these matrix proteins are required to bind the keratin filaments together and anchor them to the envelope. Adapted from Bowden *et al.* (1987)

(γ-glutamyl–ϵ-lysine link) later in terminal differentiation (upper granular layer). The matrix and the envelope-anchoring proteins are synthesised somewhat later in the keratohyalin granules (KHG) that give the granular layer its name. Profilaggrin is expressed in the larger vacuolated granules (F-KHG) and is modified both by phosphorylation, dephosphorylation and proteolysis (Dale *et al.*, 1990). It is a histidine-rich protein and has a very repetitive structure (a polyprotein) that is reflected at the gene level. The mRNA is very large (18–20 kb) and is transcribed from a gene that is only slightly larger (no introns in the coding region). The individual filaggrin units vary in size (30–50 kDa) in different species and are released in the upper granular layer, where they interact with keratin filaments. This very specific interaction is needed in order to pack and organise the filaments into the regular dense superstructure required in the corneocytes of the horny layer. Once the filaments are in this tightly packed state, the filaggrin is digested by proteases to single amino acid residues that help to maintain the water-binding characteristics of the horny layer.

Loricrin is a protein rich in glycine, serine and also cysteine residues (8%). It is synthesised in the granular layer and is associated with the smaller, dense keratohyalin granules (L-KHG). Cloning and sequencing have shown that the primary structure closely resembles the N- and C-terminal sequences of the suprabasal keratins (K1 and K10). Secondary structure predictions show that these regions can interact with one another by forming disulphide cross-linked loops. Thus loricrin is probably responsible for binding the filaments together in the corneocyte and anchoring them to the cross-linked envelope. Recent evidence also indicates that other cysteine-rich proteins are present in KHG and it seems likely that a multigene family of related matrix proteins exists. Thus, while keratin filaments are indeed important and necessary for epidermal keratinisation, they are clearly insufficient and several other structural gene products must be expressed in the correct place and at the correct time to produce a functional cornified layer.

KERATINS AND HAIR DIFFERENTIATION

During embryogenesis the hair follicle is formed from an invagination of the epidermis, creating a unique structure whose differentiation comes under the control of a complex of specialised fibroblasts, the dermal papilla. This interaction not only changes the type of structural proteins made, but also influences the changes that occur in the hair growth cycle. The bulk of the hair shaft is made from hair-specific keratin IF proteins together with several specialised matrix proteins. The terminology is confused with regard to hair keratins and it is important to distinguish between hair-specific keratin IF proteins (low-sulphur keratins) and hair matrix proteins, some of which are called high-sulphur (HS) keratins and ultra-high-sulphur (UHS) keratins (Powell and Rogers, 1986). The keratin IF proteins that are expressed in the outer root sheath of the hair follicle, the sebaceous duct and the sebaceous gland are more closely related to those of the epidermis (and other 'soft' epithelial tissues) than the hair-specific keratins themselves.

The outer root sheath (ORS) of the hair follicle expresses four keratins (K5, K6, K14, K16) and there is also some evidence for the expression of K17 in the lower parts of the ORS and sebaceous duct. The upper ORS, contiguous with the epidermis, expresses K1 and K10 suprabasally, but expression of these two keratins is reduced in the region just above the sebaceous gland. K19 expression has also been identified in the lower ORS (in the presumptive stem cell region) and in the epithelial cells of the sebaceous gland. Speculation continues on the expression of keratins in the inner root sheath (IRS), which is the site of trichohyalin synthesis (expressed in trichohyalin granules similar to keratohyalin granules of the epidermal granular cells). Expression of K6, K7, K10 and K16 has been reported in the cells of the IRS, but this is unconfirmed, as is the case for K8 and K18 expression in the lower ORS. There is also speculation as to which, if any, keratins are expressed by the epithelial cells that lie between the dermal papilla and the hair bulb trichocytes. Electron microscopy shows these cells to be virtually devoid of IF and reports of K5 and K14 expression require confirmation.

The keratin IF proteins expressed in the germinative matrix cells of the hair bulb (trichocytes), which form the filamentous component of the hair shaft, are a distinct subset of eight hair-specific keratins (Table 2.7). These keratins – the low-sulphur α-keratins of the wool literature (Tables 2.3 and 2.4), are also divided into type II basic (HaKb1–4) and type I acidic (HaKa1–4). Studies of rat tail scales, tongue epithelium and nail have identified two other closely related keratins (Hbx and Hax) which may exist as minor components of the hair.

Changes in keratin expression occur during hair differentiation. The very early matrix cells of the hair bulb, just above the dermal papilla, have few if any IF (they may express low levels of K5 and K14). However, as the cells mature, the hair-specific keratin IF genes are activated and synthesis of hair-specific keratins occurs in the keratogenous zone – the area a little above the top of the dermal papilla. This has been demonstrated by antibody staining and by *in situ* hybridisation (Fig. 2.11). As the cells move further from the dermal papilla, there is expression of the high-sulphur and ultra-high-sulphur matrix proteins, which are required to form the amorphous matrix of disulphide cross-linked filaments of the hair cortex (Powell and Rogers, 1986). Changes in keratin expression in the hair bulb also occur with the hair cycle. With the onset of catagen, hair-specific keratin gene expression stops and the bulb regresses. During telogen the bulb expresses the same keratins as the ORS and hair-specific keratin genes are not activated again until anagen.

KERATINS OF THE NAIL

Human nails are composed of a combination of 'soft' epidermal/hair follicle keratins (K5, K6, K14, K16 and K19) and 'hard' hair keratins (HaKb1–4, Hbx,

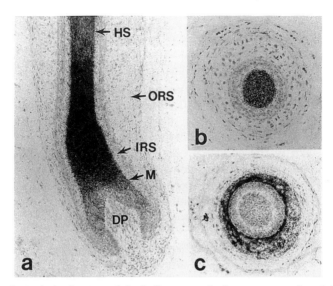

Fig. 2.11. *In situ* hybridisation of the bulk region of a human anagen hair follicle with a human type I hair-specific keratin riboprobe (a: longitudinal section; b: transverse section) and a human K14-specific riboprobe (c: transverse section). The mRNA encoding the hair keratin is localised in the keratogenous region of the hair shaft (HS) above the dermal papilla (DP). Lower matrix cells (M) show less hybridisation than the region of active hair production above. No hybridisation is seen with the hair keratin probe in the outer root sheath (ORS), inner root sheath (IRS) or the dermal papilla. In transverse sections of the bulb region (b, c), the hair keratin probe clearly hybridises to the central hair cortical cells, while the K14 probe hybridises to the ORS keratinocytes which also express K5, K6 and K16. Collaborative work with Drs G. Parker and M.B. Hodgins, University of Glasgow, UK

HaKa1–4, Hax). The epithelium of the nail plate expresses approximately 20% epidermal keratins and 80% hair keratins. In addition to this, the nail contains high-sulphur matrix proteins and possibly trichohyalin, but the exact nature of this tough, chemically resistant material is still not clear. One immunofluorescence study has shown that the epithelial cells of the ventral matrix and the nail plate have a similar pattern of keratin expression, while the apex region and the dorsal matrix are slightly different. The comparative studies available suggest that rodent claws express the same keratins, but it is not yet clear what factor(s) are responsible for maintaining the hard nature of nails and claws.

KERATINS AND EMBRYONIC DEVELOPMENT

The epidermis does not exist in the early stages (first 9 weeks) of embryonic development, and the developing fetus is covered by the periderm – a single layer of cells that contain glycogen deposits and express simple epithelial keratins (K8, K18, K19). The early epidermis develops as a single layer of basal cells with an outer periderm at about 10 weeks of fetal age, and both basal epidermal keratins (K5 and K14) and desmosomal proteins have been identified in these early keratinocytes, in addition to simple epithelial keratins. Stratification occurs at 9–14 weeks, by which time the epidermis has a layer of suprabasal cells which begin to express keratins K1 and K10, markers of epidermal differentiation. Other keratins (K4, K13, K15 and K17) have also been identified in embryonic epidermis, usually as minor components.

The dermo-epidermal junction forms at 12–14 weeks and hair follicles begin to develop at this stage. Interfollicular keratinisation begins at the 14–20-week stage, by which time a fully functional multilayered epidermis exists. At 24 weeks the epidermis expresses K1 and K10 in suprabasal cells and both K5 and K14 in basal and lower spinous cells. K6 and K16 are also expressed in the developing epidermis as well as small amounts of K8, K15, K17 and K19. By term (38–40 weeks), the epidermis has altered its expression to the adult form and only the major epidermal keratins (K1, K5, K10 and K14) are present in any quantity.

KERATIN DEFECTS AND SKIN DISEASE

Defects in skin structural proteins are thought to have a causal role in several skin disorders. Also, in skin diseases where the role of structural proteins is not central or causal, these proteins (and the genes that encode them) are useful molecular markers for the differentiation status of the epithelial cells. Among the 50 well-characterised disorders of keratinisation (see Griffiths et al., 1991), several display changes in keratin filament appearance and organisation at both light and electron microscope levels. However, specific defects in the keratins or other structural proteins were not found in early studies because the problem was not the presence or absence of a protein, or even a measurable change in size or charge, so the defects were not detected by biochemical methods. In the last few years, the application of molecular biological techniques to the characterisation of the genes that encode keratins and other major structural proteins has made it possible to study the effects of a single point mutation (a mutation which alters one base and changes one amino acid in the sequence) on keratin structure and function.

Small changes in the helical regions of a single keratin can have a dramatic effect on filament structure, as demonstrated by experiments with cellular transfection and transgenic mice. Mice which express a defective K14 gene display a disease phenotype that resembles epidermolysis bullosa simplex (EBS) – a skin condition where filament structure is disrupted and blistering results. A search for defects in K5 and K14 in families with EBS followed this preliminary evidence and now three research groups have shown that patients with EBS have mutations which are located at the ends of the helical regions (both N- and C-terminal mutations have been identified) in either K5 or K14. In one such case, a T→C mutation in exon 6 of K14 introduces a proline into the α-helical region which destabilises filament structure. These mutations are expressed in the basal cells of the epidermis, which are structurally weakened, and mechanical stress to the skin causes rupture across the basal layer resulting in blister formation. In other EBS pedigrees mutations have been found at the beginning of the 1A helix of K14 and at the end of the 2B helix in both K5 and K14 (Lane et al., 1992).

Another phenotype that has been mimicked in transgenic mice is that of epidermolytic hyperkeratosis, where introduced copies of a mutated K1 gene give rise to suprabasal keratin filament abnormalities, structural weakness of suprabasal keratinocytes and epidermal blistering. There is preliminary evidence for K1 and K10 defects in patients with epidermal hyperkeratosis, which like EBS probably results from a defective keratin gene. Hyperkeratosis has also been induced in transgenic mice by expressing a *ras* oncogene in suprabasal epidermal cells under the regulation of a K10 gene promoter, providing an *in vivo* model to study the molecular changes involved in epidermal keratinocytes by activated oncogenes.

In other disorders, where hyperproliferation of the epidermis is involved (e.g. psoriasis), altered keratin expression is probably secondary to the main cause. Whenever the epidermis is wounded, or homeostasis is lost, hyperproliferation results in a down-regulation of K1 and K10 together with an up-regulation of K6 and K16. Thus, changes in the expression of these genes are important markers of epidermal differentiation status. Finally, keratin expression also changes in skin carcinogenesis, and squamous cell carcinomas contain less K1 and K10 and more simple epithelial keratins (K8 and K18). These skin diseases are unlikely to result from primary defects of the keratin genes themselves, but alterations in their regulation may help to define the source of the molecular defects. Furthermore, keratin promoters can be used to drive the expression of various cytokines and growth modulators in cellular and transgenic systems to provide models that mimic changes in the skin of these patients.

Many of the major structural proteins of the skin have been characterised biochemically and immunologically in the last 10 years and even more recently their genes have been isolated and studied. Several other rare disorders of keratinisation must be due to defects in these same genes. Thus, in the next 5–10 years, it should be possible to elucidate the molecular mechanisms that are defective in several skin diseases, as we learn more about the function of structural proteins, the mechanisms that control cellular differentiation, and the factors involved in intracellular communication between the various cell types that make up the complex organ that we call the skin.

FUTURE RESEARCH

In the last decade a great deal of information has appeared concerning the structure, expression and regulation not only of the keratins but also of several other important structural proteins of the epidermis, hair follicle and nail. This has been fundamental to defining normal differentiation in molecular terms and has also implicated molecular defects in genetic disorders of the epidermis. The future holds even greater possibilities for a precise definition of the molecules that control cellular differentiation and further elucidation of the molecular defects behind many common skin disorders. Thus, the cell and molecular biology of the skin will form a focus for research efforts over the next decade, and if the promise of gene therapy (to correct gene defects) and genetic screening (to prevent the perpetuation of defective genes) can be fulfilled this should lead to a much lower incidence of skin disease in the future.

REFERENCES

Astbury WT and Marwick TC (1932) X-ray interpretation of the molecular structure of feather keratin. *Nature* **130**, 309–310.

Blumenberg M (1989) Evolution of homologous domains of cytoplasmic intermediate filament proteins and lamins. *Molecular Biology and Evolution* **6**, 53–65.

Bowden PE, Stark HJ, Breitkreutz D and Fusenig NE (1987) Expression and modification of keratins during terminal differentiation of mammalian epidermis. *Current Topics in Developmental Biology* **22**, 35–68.

Dale BA, Resing KA and Haydock PV (1990) Filaggrins. In: Goldman RD and Steinert PM (eds) *Cell and Molecular Biology of Intermediate Filaments*, pp. 393–412. New York: Plenum.

Franke WW, Schmid E, Schiller DL, Winter S, Jarasch ED, Moll R, Denk H, Jackson BW and Illmensee K (1982) Differentiation-related patterns of expression of proteins of intermediate-size filaments in tissues and cultured cells. *Cold Spring Harbor Symposium on Quantitative Biology* **46**, 431–453.

Gregg K and Rogers GE (1986) Feather keratin: composition, structure and biogenesis. In: Bereiter-Hahn J, Mastoltsky AG and Richards KS (eds) *Biology of the Integument*, Vol. 2: *Vertebrates*, Ch. 33, pp. 667–694. Berlin: Springer-Verlag.

Griffiths WAD, Leigh IM and Marks R (1991) Disorders of keratinisation. In: Champion RH, Burton JL and Ebling FJG (eds) *Textbook of Dermatology*, Vol. 2, 5th edn, pp. 1325–1390. Oxford: Blackwell Scientific Publications.

Heid HW, Moll I and Franke WW (1988) Patterns of expression of trichocytic and epithelial cytokeratins in mammalian tissues II. *Differentiation* **37**, 215–230.

Johnson PF and McKnight SL (1989) Eukaryotic transcriptional regulatory proteins. *Annual Review of Biochemistry* **37**, 215–230.

Krohne G and Benavente R (1986) The nuclear lamins: a multigene family of proteins in evolution and differentiation. *Experimental Cell Research* **162**, 1–10.

Lane EB, Rugg EL, Navsaria H, Leigh IM, Heagerty AHM, Ishida-Yamamoto A and Eady RAJ (1992) A mutation in the conserved helix termination peptide of keratin in hereditary skin blistering. *Nature* **356**, 244–246.

Leask A, Byrne C and Fuchs E (1991) Transcription factor AP2 and its role in epidermal-specific gene expression. *Proceedings of the National Academy of Sciences USA* **88**, 7948–7952.

Moll R, Franke WW, Schiller DL, Geiger B and Krepler R (1982) The catalog of human cytokeratins: patterns of expression in normal epithelia, tumors, and cultured cells. *Cell* **31**, 11–24.

Nagle RB (1988) Intermediate filaments: a review of the basic biology. *American Journal of Surgical Pathology* **12** (Suppl.), 4–16.

Pauling L and Corey RB (1953) Compound helical configurations of polypeptide chains: structure of proteins of the α-keratin type. *Nature* **171**, 59–61.

Popescu NC, Bowden PE and DiPaolo JA (1989) Two type II keratin genes are localised on human chromosome 12. *Human Genetics* **82**, 109–112.

Powell BC and Rogers GE (1986) Hair keratin: composition, structure and biogenesis. In: Bereiter-Hahn J, Matoltsky AG and Richards KS (eds) *Biology of the Integument*, Vol. 2: *Vertebrates*, pp. 695–721. Berlin: Springer-Verlag.

Steinert PM and Roop DR (1988) Molecular and cellular biology of intermediate filaments. *Annual Review of Biochemistry* **57**, 593–625.

Tobiasch E, Winter H and Schweizer J (1992) Structural features and site of expression of a new murine 65 kDa and 48 kDa 'hair-related' keratin pair, associated with parakeratotic epithelial differentiation. *Journal of Investigative Dermatology* **98**, 512.

BOOKS FOR REFERENCE AND FURTHER READING

Alberts B, Bray D, Lewis J, Raff M, Roberts K and Watson JD (eds) (1989) *Molecular Biology of the Cell*. New York: Garland Publishing.

Champion RH, Burton JL and Ebling FJG (eds) (1991) *Textbook of Dermatology*, 5th edn. Oxford: Blackwell Scientific Publications.

Marks R and Plewig G (eds) (1983) *Stratum Corneum*. Berlin: Springer-Verlag.

Orfanos CE and Happle R (eds) (1989) *Hair and Hair Diseases*. Berlin: Springer-Verlag.

Parry DAD and Creamer LK (eds) (1979) *Fibrous Proteins: Scientific, Industrial and Medical Aspects*. London: Academic Press.

Rogers GE, Reis PJ, Ward KA and Marshall RC (eds) (1989) *The Biology of Wool and Hair*. London: Chapman & Hall.

Sawyer RH (ed.) (1987) *Current Topics in Developmental Biology, Vol. 22: The Molecular and Developmental Biology of Keratins*. Orlando: Academic Press.

Shay JW (ed.) (1986) *Cell and Molecular Biology of the Cytoskeleton*. New York: Plenum Press.

Wang E, Fischman D, Liem RKH and Sun T-T (1985) Intermediate filaments. *Annals of the New York Academy of Sciences* **455**.

3 Skin Pigmentation and its Regulation

A.J. THODY

Protection against ultraviolet radiation (UVR) is a most important function of the skin. Although UVR has a number of beneficial effects in the skin, such as the photoconversion of 7-dehydrocholesterol into vitamin D_3, most of its effects are in fact harmful. In the short term these may be seen as sunburn reactions but following long-term exposure to UVR more serious damage can occur, including neoplastic changes. It is now recognised that UVR is a major factor in skin ageing and in the development of skin cancers, including malignant melanoma.

The skin has several mechanisms to protect against UVR-induced damage and in man one of the first lines of defence is the absorption of UVR by chromophores within the skin. A number of UV-absorbing molecules exist in the skin, including DNA, urocanic acid and amino acids. The pigment *melanin* absorbs over a broad spectrum, including UVA and UVB – the two major wavebands that reach the earth's surface. It is not a particularly efficient absorber of UV, however, and current opinion favours the idea that it photoprotects in some other way, possibly as a quencher of free radicals that are generated in response to UVR.

There are basically two types of melanins in mammals: the brownish-black *eumelanin* and the reddish-yellow *phaeomelanin*. A third group of pigments known as the trichochromes has also been found in certain types of yellow or red hair. Eumelanin is an insoluble, high-molecular-weight polymer of indole quinone and in mammals is always attached to a protein. The phaeomelanins differ from the eumelanins in that they contain a high proportion of sulphur and are soluble in dilute alkali (Prota, 1980). It is generally considered that eumelanin has the greater protective role against UVR. For a long time phaeomelanin was believed to be confined to hair but there is now evidence that both pigments are present in human skin (Thody *et al.*, 1991).

MELANOCYTES

Melanin production occurs within specialised cells in the skin known as melanocytes. These cells originate from the neural crest and during

Molecular Aspects of Dermatology. Edited by G.C. Priestley.
© 1993 by John Wiley & Sons Ltd

embryogenesis migrate to various sites throughout the body, including the skin (Rawles, 1947). Within the skin they become associated either with the hair follicles or the basal layer of the epidermis. Epidermal melanocytes are thin, elongated cells with long dendritic processes which ramify among neighbouring epidermal cells (Fig. 3.1). This facilitates the transfer of melanosomes to the keratinocytes and in this way melanin is distributed into the suprabasal regions of the epidermis, where it protects the germinative cells of the basal layer from UVR. In the human epidermis each melanocyte is normally associated with approximately 36 keratinocytes and together they constitute the epidermal melanin unit (Fitzpatrick and Breathnach, 1963). Although melanocyte density varies quite considerably in different regions of the human skin, the total number is relatively constant, even in different racial groups. The average density is in the range 1000–2000 melanocytes/cm^2 skin.

In some mammals melanocytes are also found in the dermis. These melanocytes, unlike their epidermal counterparts, seem unable to secrete their pigment granules; because of this and their position in the dermis they would seem to have no role in protecting the skin from the harmful effects of UV. However, by affecting the refraction of light, the dermal melanocytes can influence skin colour and in some primates, e.g. certain Old World monkeys, this may be important in social and sexual communication.

Skin pigmentation depends upon the organisation and functioning of the epidermal melanin unit and six separate but related events: (1) melanoblast migration from the neural crest; (2) melanoblast differentiation into melanocytes; (3) melanosome formation; (4) melanin synthesis; (5) melanin transfer from the melanocyte into keratinocytes; and (6) melanosome degradation within the keratinocytes.

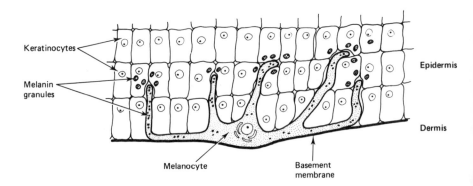

Fig. 3.1. Epidermal melanocytes are situated on the basement membrane. Melanin is formed within these cells and transferred into the neighbouring keratinocytes via the dendritic processes. Each melanocyte is normally associated with 36 keratinocytes and together the cells form the epidermal melanin unit. Reproduced from Thody and Friedmann (1986) by permission of Churchill Livingstone

MELANOCYTE DEVELOPMENT

This process has been well studied in mice. Melanoblast determination becomes active at about days 5–7 of gestation, and between days 8 and 12 the melanoblasts migrate from the neural crest to the skin. Melanocyte differentiation then takes place and on the 15th day of gestation the melanocytes contain developing melanosomes. The melanocytes increase in number until day 3 postpartum, after which there is a gradual decline. Less is known about the development of human melanocytes, but migration from the neural crest occurs at around week 8 of fetal life. There is also a reduction in melanocyte numbers following parturition but whether this represents a real loss or simply a conversion to amelanotic or resting melanocytes is not yet clear.

Little is known about the mechanisms that regulate melanoblast migration. It is, however, recognised that the c-kit gene is highly expressed on melanoblasts during this migratory phase and persists following their colonisation of the skin. In mice c-kit maps to the W locus on chromosome 5 and has recently been shown to code for a transmembrane receptor with tyrosine kinase activity. Mutations at the W locus reduce the numbers of melanocytes developing in the skin and this results in white spotting of the hair or, in extreme cases, a complete loss of hair pigmentation. Other developmental processes such as haematopoiesis and germ cell formation are also affected. These same processes are disrupted by mutations at the steel locus and it appears that this locus encodes for a factor, variously known as steel factor (SLF), kit ligand (KL), stem cell factor (SCF) or mast cell growth factor (MGF), that serves as the ligand for the c-kit product.

MELANOSOME FORMATION

The melanosomes are the intracellular site of melanin synthesis. These subcellular organelles arise from the endoplasmic reticulum and are first recognised as spherical, membrane-coated vesicles (Fig. 3.2). Their protein structure becomes organised into a matrix of filaments and at this stage, if the organelles are destined to become eumelanosomes, they assume an elliptical shape. Phaeomelanosomes, on the other hand, maintain their spherical shape throughout and, unlike the eumelanosomes, develop no organised filamentous protein matrix. This internal structure of the melanosome becomes obscured as melanin is synthesised and deposited. Tyrosinase, the enzyme that initiates melanin synthesis, becomes incorporated into the melanosome during this period of development (see later). Presumably the same occurs with other enzymes, e.g. dopachrome tautomerase, that are involved in regulating melanin synthesis.

MELANOGENESIS

The initial steps in the synthesis of eumelanin and phaeomelanin are under the control of the enzyme tyrosinase, which oxidises tyrosine to 3,4-dihydro-

Melanocyte   Keratinocyte

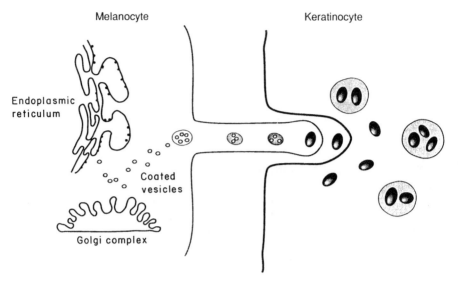

Endoplasmic
reticulum

Coated
vesicles

Golgi complex

Fig. 3.2. Melanosome formation and transfer. The melanosomes arise from the dilated tubules of the endoplasmic reticulum. Tyrosinase, which is synthesised by the ribosomes, is incorporated into coated vesicles in the Golgi complex, and transported in this way to the developing melanosome. As the melanosomes mature they migrate to the tip of the dendritic process and are then transferred into the keratinocyte

xyphenylalanine (dopa) and then to dopaquinone (Fig. 3.3). Dopaquinone is then converted by a series of complex reactions involving cyclisation and oxidative polymerisations which finally result in the formation of eumelanin. It was once thought that these latter reactions occurred spontaneously but it appears that certain steps are under a regulatory control. For instance, there is now evidence that dopachrome can be converted to either 5,6-dihydroxyindole or the carboxy derivative 5,6-dihydroxyindole carboxylic acid (DHICA). This latter step appears to be catalysed by a recently discovered enzyme, dopachrome tautomerase, or by metal ions.

According to Prota (1980), all that is required to switch the synthetic pathway from eumelanin to phaeomelanin is the presence of sulphydryl residues. Thus if dopachrome encounters either cysteine or glutathione, cysteinyl dopas are formed, which are then quickly oxidised into benzothiazines and thence into phaeomelanins (Fig. 3.3). The cysteinyl dopas could also arise from glutathione dopa formed from a reaction between dopaquinone and glutathione. This reaction is catalysed by α-glutamyl transferase, which has been shown to be present in melanogenic melanocytes. Glutathione may have a regulatory role in melanogenesis because unless the glutathione is hydrolysed to cysteinyl dopa its formation would result in the side-tracking of the dopaquinone (Prota, 1980). It is therefore interesting that glutathione and glutathione reductase levels appear to be lower in Negroid

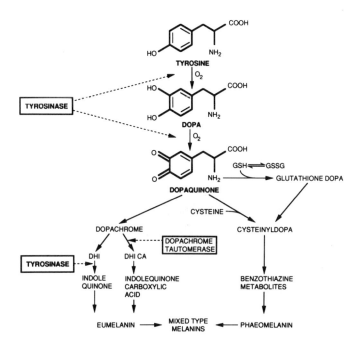

Fig. 3.3. The melanin pathway, showing the points of action of tyrosinase and dopachrome tautomerase

skin than in Caucasian skin and have also been found to be reduced following UV irradiation.

MELANOSOME MOVEMENT

This process is poorly understood. Virtually all our knowledge of melanosome movement has come from studies in fish and amphibia, where it forms the basis of the rapid colour changes characteristic of these lower vertebrates.

MELANOSOME TRANSFER

The mechanism of melanosome transfer from the dendritic processes of the melanocyte into the keratinocyte is also poorly understood (Fig. 3.2). There are at least three possibilities: (1) the keratinocytes may engulf and phagocytose the melanosome-laden dendritic tips of the melanocyte; (2) a direct uptake of melanosomes may take place through localised cell membrane fusions occurring between melanocytes and keratinocytes; and (3) melanosomes are first secreted into the intercellular spaces and then subsequently phagocytosed by the keratinocytes. All three processes may operate and this could explain why melanosomes can occur in keratinocytes either as single particles or in aggregates of two or more.

MELANOSOME DEGRADATION

Once inside the keratinocyte the melanosomes become associated with lysosomal enzymes. Negroid melanosomes are larger than those of Caucasians and this may contribute to their differences in skin colour.

TYROSINASE

Tyrosinase is the rate-limiting enzyme in the melanin pathway. It is a multifunctional copper-containing glycoprotein with a molecular size of 60–70 kDa (Fig. 3.4) (Hearing and Jiménez, 1987). In mammals it is found exclusively in melanocytes and is therefore a good specific marker for these cells.

As well as initiating melanogenesis by hydroxylating tyrosine to dopa, tyrosinase also catalyses the conversion of dopa to dopaquinone. Interestingly the initial product, dopa, also functions as a co-factor for the first reaction. Evidence suggests that it may also catalyse later steps in the eumelanin pathway, i.e. the oxidation of 5,6-dihydroxyindole to indole 5,6-quinone (Fig. 3.3).

Recently, both mouse and human tyrosinase genes have been cloned and sequenced. Tyrosinase maps to the *albino* (c) locus, which in mice is present on chromosome 7 and in humans on chromosome 11. A single point mutation, resulting in a change of a conserved cysteine at residue 85 to a serine in the tyrosinase sequence, is responsible for the albino phenotype, and all strains of albino mice so far examined have this same mutation. In recent studies it has been possible to rescue the albino phenotype in transgenic mice carrying a functional tyrosinase minigene (Beermann *et al.*, 1990; Tanaka *et al.*, 1990).

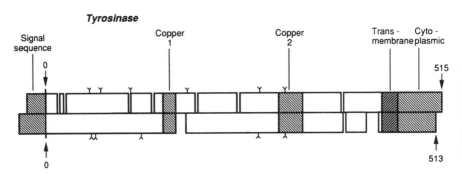

Fig. 3.4. The amino acid sequences of mouse tyrosinase and tyrosinase-related protein 1 (TRP-1). Both proteins have many common features, including two copper-binding sites and numerous glycosylation sites (Y)

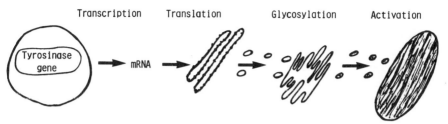

Fig. 3.5. Potential control points in the regulation of tyrosinase

Using *in situ* hybridisation, expression of the transgene was found in the melanocytes of the hair bulb and in the pigmented cells of the eye.

Transcription of the tyrosinase gene results in the formation of a protein with a molecular weight of 55 kDa, which then undergoes post-translational processing to produce several different isozymes. Glycosylation of the enzyme occurs during this post-translational processing with the addition of sialic acid and several neutral sugars, which increases the molecular weight to about 70 kDa. This post-translational glycosylation of tyrosinase occurs as the enzyme is transferred through the Golgi complex to the melanosome, where it becomes functionally active and where melanogenesis takes place.

There are therefore a number of potential control points in the regulation of tyrosinase (Fig. 3.5), involving changes in its rate of synthesis, post-translational processing, and degradation. Most studies on the control of tyrosinase have been carried out on melanoma cells where *de novo* synthesis of the enzyme and post-translational activation appear to be important regulatory steps. We have little information on the control mechanisms operating in normal melanocytes, although recent evidence suggests that in man the levels of tyrosinase synthesis vary with skin type and correlate with the ability to produce melanin. On the other hand, it has been reported that tyrosinase activity in black skin is approximately three times higher than that of white skin and that this occurs, not as a result of an increase in tyrosinase synthesis, but by a change in the catalytic activity of the enzyme. This difference could result from (1) the presence of tyrosinase inhibitors, (2) differences in the post-translational processing of the enzyme, or (3) the production of alternatively spliced tyrosinase mRNA transcripts resulting in the synthesis of different forms of tyrosinase. Although alternative splicing of tyrosinase mRNA has been shown to occur, there is currently little evidence to suggest that such processes, or differences in the rates of transcription of the tyrosinase gene, participate in the regulation of tyrosinase.

TYROSINASE-RELATED PROTEINS

During studies aimed at cloning the tyrosinase gene, several other tyrosinase-related proteins (TRP genes) were also inadvertently cloned. The first of these, designated pMT4, was cloned from mouse melanoma cDNA using monoclonal anti-tyrosinase antibodies. Although this was originally thought to be tyrosinase cDNA, it did not confer tyrosinase activity on transfected cells and was subsequently mapped to the brown (b) locus of mice rather than the c locus (Jackson, 1988). The encoded product does, nevertheless, show high homology to tyrosinase and for this reason has been designated tyrosinase-related protein 1 (TRP-1) (Fig. 3.4). A second tyrosinase-related protein (TRP-2) has been mapped to the slaty locus and a third (Pmel17) to the silver locus in mice.

The functions of these different proteins are not yet known. There are reports that TRP-1 has catalase activity or, alternatively, a role in regulating the activity of tyrosinase. TRP-2, on the other hand, is thought to be dopachrome tautomerase, the enzyme which isomerises dopachrome to DHICA (see above). Korner and Pawelek (1980) were the first to suggest the presence of a dopachrome conversion factor, but it was realised later that the product of this reaction was DHICA. The purification of dopachrome tautomerase has proved difficult and molecular weight estimates have varied considerably. A major problem is that dopachrome tautomerase co-purifies with tyrosinase and may exist in a complex with tyrosinase, TRP-1 and possibly other proteins such as the melanocyte-stimulating hormone (MSH) receptor.

The biological significance of dopachrome tautomerase is also not yet clear. One possibility is that it may determine the type of melanin that is produced within the melanocytes. Thus DHICA-derived melanins are brown in appearance and are different from the black melanins that are produced from DHI. Increases in the activity of dopachrome tautomerase might therefore lead to the production of brown rather than black melanins. DHICA is also relatively less toxic than DHI, and for this reason dopachrome tautomerase may have an important role in reducing the cytotoxic effects arising from the synthesis of melanin.

Thus it is beginning to emerge that, in addition to tyrosinase, numerous other gene products function in controlling mammalian melanogenesis and may regulate not only the amount but also the type of melanin that is produced within the melanocyte.

REGULATION OF SKIN PIGMENTATION

Skin pigmentation can be considered to consist of two components. The first, *constitutive pigmentation*, is the pigmentation which is genetically determined in the absence of stimulatory influences, i.e. the level of pigmentation in parts of the body that are not normally exposed to UVR. The second, *facultative pigmentation*, is the level of pigmentation or tanning that occurs in response to stimulatory influences. In man, facultative skin pigmentation can be induced by two major factors: UVR and hormones (Fig. 3.6).

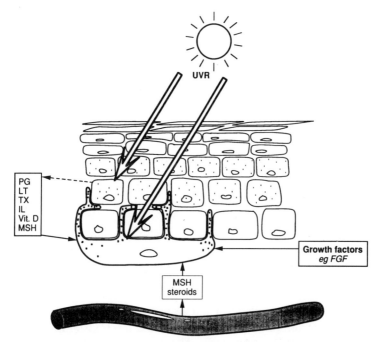

Fig. 3.6. Factors involved in the regulation of melanocytes. FGF, basic fibroblast growth factor; IL, interleukins; LT, leukotrienes; MSH, melanocyte-stimulating hormone; PG, prostaglandins; TX, thromboxanes; UVR, ultraviolet radiation; Vit D, vitamin D_3

EFFECT OF UV RADIATION

In man, sunlight is probably the most important physiological stimulator of the pigmentary system and is responsible for bringing about the normal tanning response. The solar radiation that reaches the earth's surface can be divided into UVB (290–320 nm), UVA (320–380 nm), visible light (380–760 nm) and near-infrared (> 760 nm). Although wavelengths in the visible region have been shown to induce photobiological effects, it is the UV spectrum that causes the tanning response in the skin. This tanning involves two distinct reactions. The first, or immediate reaction, which occurs within a few minutes of exposure to UVA and lasts for up to 4 hours, is characterised by the photo-oxidation of pre-formed melanin. There have been suggestions that the melanosomes move towards the dendritic processes of the melanocyte, with an increase in their numbers in the keratinocytes. However, others have failed to confirm these ultrastructural changes.

The delayed action which occurs in response to both UVA and UVB is much slower in onset and is only apparent after 2–3 days of repeated exposure. This delayed response involves an increase in the numbers of active melanocytes,

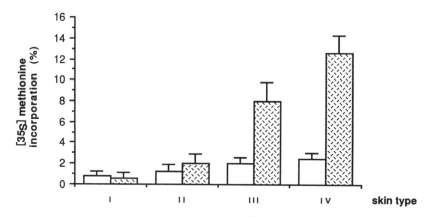

Fig. 3.7. Tyrosinase synthesis (as measured by the incorporation of [^{35}S]methionine) in skin biopsies from different skin types before (unshaded) and after (shaded) PUVA (psoralen UVA) therapy

enhanced melanosome production and an increase in melanogenesis. There is also an increase in keratinocyte proliferation and the transfer of melanosomes from the melanocytes into these cells. The increased numbers of melanocytes result from an enhanced proliferation and also possibly from an activation of precursor amelanotic melanocytes. UVR also stimulates the synthesis of tyrosinase (Fig. 3.7) and this is followed by melanisation of the melanosomes. It is not yet known how UVR acts on the melanocytes to induce both proliferation and an increase in melanogenesis and it seems likely that different signals are involved. These could result from a direct action of UVR on the melanocytes and through indirect actions on other cells such as keratinocytes. As discussed below, there is now much evidence that keratinocytes are responsible for a number of substances that can affect both melanocyte growth and melanogenesis.

The ability to tan in response to UV does, however, vary in different individuals and on the basis of this tanning response it is possible to identify different skin types (Table 3.1). The mechanisms underlying these differences in tanning response are not yet fully understood. One possibility is a differential expression of the tyrosinase gene, and although this has not yet

Table 3.1. Skin types

Skin type	History
I	Always burns, never tans
II	Always burns, sometimes tans
III	Sometimes burns, always tans
IV	Never burns, always tans

been examined, tyrosinase synthesis has been shown to correlate positively with tanning ability (Fig. 3.7). Persons with skin type I, who always burn in response to UV and never tan, are the most susceptible to UV-induced skin damage, including skin cancers. This is thought to depend upon the amount of melanin in the skin but the type of melanin could also be important. Thus phaeomelanin, which is now known to be present in human skin, has a greater capacity to produce free radicals in response to UVR and, since these are capable of inflicting cell injury, phaeomelanin may actually contribute to UV-induced skin damage, rather than protecting the skin.

EFFECT OF THE LOCAL ENVIRONMENT

It has been known for a long time that a functional relationship exists between melanocytes and neighbouring keratinocytes. The keratinocytes, as well as receiving melanosomes from the melanocyte, appear to play an important role in regulating melanocyte growth and differentiation (De Luca et al., 1988). The identity of the keratinocyte-derived substances that influence melanocyte behaviour is still not clear although there are several possible candidates (Fig. 3.6).

One candidate is basic fibroblast growth factor (bFGF). This substance is produced by several different cells, including keratinocytes and fibroblasts, and may be a natural melanocyte mitogen acting in a paracrine manner to regulate melanocyte growth (Halaban et al., 1987). Other members of the FGF family and other growth factors such as mast cell growth factor (MGF) and hepatocyte growth factor (HGF) also act as melanocyte mitogens and may be produced in the skin.

When human melanocytes are cultured with keratinocytes they express dendrites that make contact with the keratinocytes, as seen in vivo. It appears that the keratinocytes produce factors that stimulate melanocyte dendricity. Keratinocytes also produce numerous other factors, including cytokines, eicosanoids and vitamin D_3, many of which have been reported to affect melanocyte growth and/or melanogenesis. The skin is also a source of MSH and there is evidence that this is produced by keratinocytes. UVR causes the release of some of these factors and perhaps they mediate some of the effects that UV has on melanocytes. Post-inflammatory pigmentation might also depend on locally produced chemical mediators.

Certain cytokines that are produced by keratinocytes, e.g. tumour necrosis factor α (TNFα), interleukin 1α (IL-1α) and interferons, have been shown to induce the expression of the intercellular adhesion molecule 1 (ICAM-1) on cultured human melanocytes (Yohn et al., 1990). Since ICAM-1 is the ligand for leucocyte function associated antigen (LFA-1), its expression on melanocytes could suggest a role for these cells in cutaneous immunological reactions and inflammatory responses. Further support for this hypothesis is the recent evidence that melanocytes can secrete several different cytokines. However, it remains to be shown that human melanocytes *in vivo* have these properties.

Within the skin, epidermal melanocytes are normally associated with the basement membrane. The basement membrane not only serves as a substratum for the melanocytes but could also play an active part in regulating melanocyte behaviour. Extracellular matrix (ECM) proteins, such as fibronectin and laminin, facilitate melanocyte attachment, influence cell morphology and may also regulate pigment cell migration, but little is known of the mechanisms involved.

HORMONAL CONTROL

Melanocytes respond to many hormonal stimuli, and the two most important groups in this respect are the MSH peptides and sex steroids (Fig. 3.6).

The MSH peptides

Administration of MSH produces darkening of the skin and hair in numerous mammalian species. Lerner and McGuire (1961) were the first to demonstrate that MSH peptides darken human skin, and Levine and associates (1991) have recently confirmed these findings using a potent analogue of α-MSH. It is interesting that the greatest tanning was seen in sun-exposed areas and this could indicate a synergistic effect of sunlight and MSH.

There are several MSH peptides. They are produced mainly in the pituitary gland together with adrenocorticotrophic hormone (ACTH), lipotrophin (LPH), and the endorphins from the same 31 kDa precursor protein proopiomelanocortin (POMC). Although POMC is synthesised in both the pars anterior and the pars intermedia, it is processed differently in these two lobes. In the former it is cleaved to give ACTH and LPH, but in the pars intermedia these peptides are further cleaved to give either α-MSH and CLIP (corticotrophin-like intermediate lobe peptide) or β-MSH and β-endorphin respectively. It was once believed that the main pigmentary hormone in man was the 22 amino acid β-MSH but it is now thought that this particular peptide was an extraction artefact and that the human immunoreactive β-MSH is probably due to LPH. The human pituitary, in contrast to that of other mammals, has a poorly developed intermediate lobe and it appears that the main pigmentary hormones produced by the human pituitary are ACTH and LPH. Increased secretion of these peptides may be responsible for the hyperpigmentation associated with a number of endocrinopathies, e.g. Addison's disease. In certain circumstances the human pituitary may also produce α-MSH, which could contribute to any hyperpigmentation that occurs. An intermediate lobe is present in the fetal human pituitary and this seems to be capable of producing α-MSH. Whether α-MSH has a role in the development of the pigmentary system remains to be seen.

The pituitary is not the only site of MSH production: MSH peptides are produced in other sites, including the skin (Thody *et al.*, 1983). This locally produced MSH may well participate in regulating melanocytes (see above) and could also have other roles in the skin. For instance, it is now established that α-MSH has anti-inflammatory activity and may well act as a modulator of the immune system. In this connection it is interesting that melanocytes may have a role in mediating immunological reactions (see above).

Steroids

Ovarian steroids increase skin pigmentation in guinea-pigs. Testosterone, on the other hand, appears to have no pigmentary effects in the guinea-pig, although androgens increase skin pigmentation in other species. In rats, testosterone increases tyrosinase activity in scrotal melanocytes. The effects of adrenal steroids have received less attention, though there are reports that they have no pigmentary effects in male guinea-pigs.

Increased pigmentation of the nipples, areola, face, abdominal skin and genitalia is often seen in pregnant women. These changes are similar to those produced by oestrogens and progesterone in the guinea-pig and these steroids are thought to be responsible for the pigmentary changes in pregnancy and also the melasma sometimes seen in women taking oral contraceptives. Melasma is the hyperpigmentation which occurs on the face and other sun-exposed areas. This distribution suggests an interaction between steroids and solar radiation, but this has yet to confirmed.

TRANSMEMBRANE AND INTRACELLULAR PATHWAYS

Several different signal transduction pathways operate in pigment cells (Fig. 3.8), the best known being the adenylate cyclase/cyclic AMP (cAMP) system. MSH is a well-known activator of this system in melanoma cells and mouse hair follicular melanocytes. The initial event involves the binding of the peptide to specific cell surface receptors, and this leads to an activation of adenylate cyclase via the stimulatory guanine nucleotide binding protein (Gs). The activated adenylate cyclase then catalyses the synthesis of cAMP from ATP and after a lag period of 6–9 hours there is an increase in tyrosinase activity. The events during this period are not understood but, by analogy with other cAMP-mediated responses, it would appear that a cAMP-dependent protein kinase is activated, leading to an increase in protein synthesis. In some melanocytes tyrosinase itself is synthesised, although pre-existing tyrosinase molecules may also be activated. Whatever the mechanism, the consequence is an increase in melanogenesis. Although human melanocytes express specific and high-affinity MSH receptors, there are reports that cultured human melanocytes show only small increases in cAMP in response to α-MSH. This may explain why several authors have failed to observe melanogenic effects with α-MSH in human melanocytes *in vitro*.

Activation of adenylate cyclase also increases melanocyte proliferation and

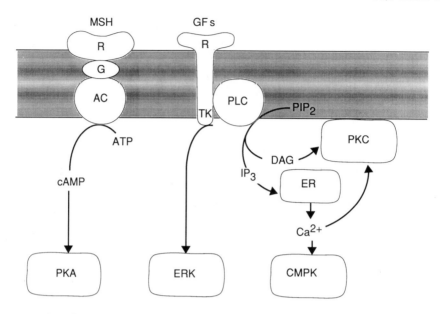

Fig. 3.8. Possible hormone and growth factor-activated signalling pathways in pigment cells. The interaction of a hormone, such as MSH, with its receptor (R) in the cell membrane promotes the activation of the stimulatory G protein (G), which in turn activates adenylate cylase (AC) and this generates the formation of cAMP, which then phosphorylates the cAMP-dependent protein kinase (PKA). Growth factors (GFs), on the other hand, interact with their receptors to bring about the activation of a tyrosine kinase (TK), which phosphorylates several different substrates including the early response kinase (ERK) and a phospholipase (PLC). The latter hydrolyses phosphatidylinositol 4,5-bisphosphate (PIP_2), generating two second messengers: diacylglycerol (DAG), which activates protein kinase C (PKC) and inositol 1,4,5-trisphosphate (IP_3), which triggers the release of Ca^{2+} from intracellular stores such as the endoplasmic reticulum (ER). An associated stimulation of Ca^{2+} entry across the plasma membrane may also occur (not shown). By activating the calmodulin-dependent protein kinase (CMPK), Ca^{2+} may inhibit melanogenesis and in this way oppose the stimulatory action of cAMP

for this reason agents that elevate cAMP, e.g. choleratoxin, are often included in melanocyte culture systems. Growth factors, such as bFGF, MGF and HGF, also stimulate melanocyte proliferation and synergise with cAMP to bring about this response. Rather than activating adenylate cyclase, these growth factors stimulate receptors with tyrosine kinase (TK) activity and this brings about the phosphorylation of a variety of substrates. In human melanocytes one such phosphorylated intermediate has been identified as the early response kinase (ERK) or mitogen-activated protein (MAP) kinase (Funasaka *et al.*, 1992). Other possible substrates for activated TK include a phospholipase (PLC) which, when activated, hydrolyses phosphatidylinositol 4,5-bisphosphate (PIP_2) with the formation of two second messengers, inositol 1,4,5-trisphosphate (IP_3) and diacylglycerol (DAG).

DAG, which activates protein kinase C (PKC), has been shown to stimulate melanogenesis in human melanocytes and melanoma cells. Phorbol 12-myristate 13-acetate (TPA), however, also activates PKC but appears to have little or no effect on melanogenesis. On the other hand, the phorbol ester is a potent mitogen for human melanocytes. Thus while PKC clearly has an important role in the melanocyte, its precise function is still unknown. IP_3, the other second messenger formed from PIP_2, induces the release of calcium from intracellular stores. Mobilisation of Ca^{2+} may also occur as a result of entry via calcium channels in the plasma membrane. Calcium has an important role in the regulation of the melanocyte. For instance, there is evidence in mouse melanoma cells that calcium serves as a second messenger in the regulation of melanogenesis, but rather than stimulating this process it appears to have an inhibitory action. Since antagonists of the calcium binding protein, calmodulin, have the opposite effect and stimulate melanogenesis, the possibility exists that the inhibitory action of calcium involves an activation of a calmodulin-dependent protein kinase. It is clear that we still have much to learn about the intracellular mechanisms that operate in melanocytes and their role in regulating growth and differentiation.

PIGMENTARY DISORDERS

As described earlier in this chapter, skin pigmentation is the end product of a complex but interrelated series of morphological and biochemical processes involving the migration and differentiation of melanoblasts, the synthesis of malanosomes and melanin, the transfer of melanosomes to keratinocytes and their subsequent degradation. Many, if not all, these processes are genetically controlled and are also influenced by extrinsic factors such as UVR and hormones. The different processes in this multistep pathway are closely integrated and a defect at any one stage is likely to disrupt the subsequent steps. It is therefore often difficult to classify pigmentary disorders on the basis of a primary defect.

There are, however, several disorders where the primary defect can be identified. For instance, *piebaldism* can be explained on the basis of a defect in melanoblast migration and development. It appears that although melanoblasts enter the skin they fail to survive at their most distant sites. This results in an area of unpigmented skin in the anterior midline which is the basis for the most characteristic feature of piebaldism, i.e. the white forelock. Animal models of piebaldism exist. Thus, as described earlier, white spotting of the hair occurs in mice bearing mutations at the W or *steel* locus. These mutations affect the function of a growth factor receptor and as a result the melanoblasts fail to proliferate. Whether similar mutations exist in human piebaldism is not yet established.

Melanocytic naevi can also result from disturbances in the migration and/or differentiation of melanoblasts. During their migration to the epidermis of the hair follicles, some melanoblasts remain in the dermis where they mature. This results in the *Mongolian blue spot*, which can be single or multiple. A more localised accumulation of melanocytes, together with related naevus cells, can also occur. These are sometimes found in the lower layers of the dermis but are more common in the superficial dermis and epidermis, where they form what is known as the *compound naevus*. If present at the dermal/epidermal junction they are referred to as *junctional naevi*. These lesions appear during the first few years of life, but new ones may continue to develop throughout the first two decades. When present at birth they can be much larger and more bizarre in appearance. The naevus cells within these lesions, like melanocytes, are derived from the neural crest. They also contain tyrosinase and primary melanosomes but their melanin content varies greatly. Thus naevocytic naevi can show varying degrees of melanisation.

Increased numbers of melanocytes at the dermal/epidermal junction are also seen in disorders characterised as *lentigines*. These lesions are thought to result from an increase in the proportion of metabolically active melanocytes. The *ephelides* or *freckles* that are commonly seen in people with blue eyes and red or blonde hair are not due to an increase in melanocyte numbers, but are thought to represent areas of increased melanin synthesis. The melanocytes and keratinocytes present in these lesions contain large dark oval eumelanomones like those in dark-skinned people, whereas in the pale skin that exists between the freckles the melanocytes contain smaller round phaeomelanosomes. Freckles appear in childhood and their number and degree of pigmentation usually increase during summer, indicating that the melanocytes respond to UV.

Café au lait spots also contain melanocytes that are hyperactive. Increased numbers of melanosomes are present in these cells, together with giant melanosomes which are also present in keratinocytes. Café au lait spots have a well-defined border and are over 1.5 cm in size. The presence of five or more such patches in a patient is said to indicate *neurofibromatosis*, a condition characterised by abnormalities in the differentiation of other neural crest elements such as Schwann cells. The defective gene in patients with neurofibromatosis has recently been identified and its product, known as neurofibromin, is a GTPase-activating protein (GAP) that regulates the activity of the *ras* proto-oncogene product. Café au lait spots are also seen in the *McCune–Albright syndrome* which, like neurofibromatosis, also involves multiple abnormalities. Recent evidence suggests that this syndrome is the result of a mutation in the Gs protein and this, by reducing the protein's intrinsic GTPase activity, causes persistent activation of adenylate cyclase leading to an increased level of cAMP. This presumably accounts for the increased melanogenic activity of the melanocytes in this syndrome since, as discussed earlier, cAMP is an important second messenger system in pigment cells.

Endocrine disorders involving increased secretion of peptides such as MSH or ACTH may also cause changes in pigmentation due to an activation of adenylate cyclase (see above). The hyperpigmentation that occurs in certain endocrinopathies where there is increased secretion of ACTH and MSH, e.g. *Addison's disease* – ectopic ACTH syndrome – is also likely to be the result of an increase in adenylate cyclase activity in the melanocyte. However, the pigmentation in these conditions is generally diffuse and is not confined to circumscribed pigmentary lesions as seen in neurofibromatosis and the McCune–Albright syndrome. The reason for this is not entirely clear. It could be that in the endocrine-related pigmentary conditions the pigmentation results from the changes induced by the circulating hormones and, unlike the aforementioned disorders, there is no intrinsic abnormality within the melanocyte.

Albinism is a good example of a pigmentary disorder involving a disruption of melanin synthesis. There are several different types of albinism, each involving a change in the function of tyrosinase – the enzyme that controls the initial steps in the melanin pathway (see earlier). In *tyrosinase-negative albinism*, where there is a total loss of pigmentation in all tissues, there is a failure in the synthesis of the tyrosinase enzyme. In *tyrosinase-positive albinism* it appears that some residual tyrosinase activity remains and some melanin pigment is formed in the eyes, skin and hair. During the first years of life this is predominantly of the phaeomelanin type but is then followed by eumelanin synthesis in the adult. These two types of albinism appear to result from different mutations at a single locus. Other types of oculo-cutaneous albinism can arise through defects in the disruption of melanosome formation and transfer to keratinocytes. For example, in the *Chediak–Higashi syndrome* the melanocytes contain giant melanosomes which appear to be too large to transfer into the keratinocytes. Hypopigmentation of the skin is also seen in *phenylketonuria*. In this condition there is a reduced availability of tyrosine, due to a deficiency of hepatic phenylalanine hydroxylase which converts phenylalanine, derived from dietary protein, to tyrosine. Administration of tyrosine will increase skin pigmentation in this condition.

The number of melanocytes in the skin will clearly have an important bearing upon the level of pigmentation. In certain disorders, such as *vitiligo*, epidermal melanocytes are destroyed, resulting in patches of depigmentation. The mechanisms responsible for this melanocyte destruction are not yet clear. One possibility is a breakdown in immune surveillance which affects melanocyte function and subsequently its destruction. The neural hypothesis proposes that a neurochemical mediator is responsible for the destruction of the melanocytes or inhibits their ability to produce melanin. In the self-destruction hypothesis, it has been suggested that these same effects are brought about by metabolic products of melanin synthesis. None of these theories is entirely satisfactory and there may be a number of different causes for this hypopigmentary disorder.

REFERENCES

Beermann F, Ruppert S, Hummler E, Bosch FX, Müller G, Rüther U and Schütz G (1990) Rescue of the albino phenotype by introduction of a functional tyrosinase gene into mice. *EMBO Journal* **9**, 2819–2826.

De Luca M, D'Anna F, Bondanza S, Franzi AT and Cancedda R (1988) Human epithelial cells induce human melanocyte growth in vitro but only skin keratinocytes regulate its proper differentiation in the absence of dermis. *Journal of Cell Biology* **107**, 1919–1926.

Fitzpatrick TB and Breathnach AS (1963) Das epidermale melanin Einheit system. *Dermatologische Wochenschrift* **147**, 481–489.

Funasaka Y, Boulton T, Cobb M, Yarden Y, Fan B, Lyman SD, Williams DE, Anderson DM, Zakut R, Mishima Y and Halaban R (1992) c-kit-kinase induces a cascade of protein tyrosine phosphorylation in normal human melanocytes in response to mast cell growth factor and stimulates mitogen-activated protein kinase but is down-regulated in melanomas. *Molecular Biology of the Cell* **3**, 197–209.

Halaban R, Ghosh S and Baird A (1987) bFGF is the putative natural growth factor for human melanocytes. *In Vitro Cellular and Developmental Biology* **23**, 47–52.

Hearing VJ and Jiménez M (1987) Mammalian tyrosinase: the critical regulatory control point in melanocyte pigmentation. *International Journal of Biochemistry* **19**, 1141–1147.

Jackson I (1988) A cDNA encoding tyrosinase related protein maps to the mouse brown locus. *Proceedings of the National Academy of Sciences USA* **85**, 4392–4396.

Korner AM and Pawelek JM (1980) Dopamine conversion: a possible control point in melanin biosynthesis. *Journal of Investigative Dermatology* **75**, 192–195.

Lerner AB and McGuire JS (1961) Effect of alpha- and beta-melanocyte stimulating hormones on the skin colour of man. *Nature* **189**, 176–179.

Levine N, Sheftel SN, Eytan T, Dorr RT, Hadley ME, Weinrach JC, Ertl GA, Toth K, McGee DL and Hruby VJ (1991). Induction of skin tanning by subcutaneous administration of a potent synthetic melanotropin. *Journal of the American Medical Association* **266**, 2730–2736.

Prota G (1980) Recent advances in the chemistry of melanogenesis in mammals. *Journal of Investigative Dermatology* **75**, 122–127.

Rawles ME (1947) Origin of pigment cells from the neural crest in the mouse embryo. *Physiological Zoology* **20**, 248–266.

Tanaka S, Yamamoto H, Takeuchi S and Takeuchi T (1990) Melanization in albino mice transformed by introducing cloned mouse tyrosinase gene. *Development* **108**, 223–227.

Thody AJ, Ridley K, Penny RJ, Chalmers R, Fisher C and Shuster S (1983) MSH peptides are present in mammalian skin. *Peptides* **4**, 813–816.

Thody AJ, Higgins EM, Wakamatsu K, Ito S, Burchill SA and Marks JM (1991) Phaeomelanin as well as eumelanin is present in human epidermis. *Journal of Investigative Dermatology* **97**, 340–334.

Yohn JJ, Critelli M, Lyons MB and Norris DA (1990) Modulation of melanocyte intercellular adhesion molecule-1 by immune cytokines. *Journal of Investigative Dermatology* **90**, 233–237.

FURTHER READING

Bennett DC (1991) Colour genes, oncogenes and melanocyte differentiation. *Journal of Cell Science* **98**, 135–139.

Eberle A (1988) *The Melanotropins: Chemistry, Physiology and Mechanisms of Action.* Basel: Karger.

Fitzpatrick TB, Pathak MA, Harber LC, Seiji M and Kukita A (eds) (1974) *Normal and Abnormal Photobiologic Responses*. Tokyo: University of Tokyo Press.

Halaban R (1991) Growth factors regulating normal and malignant melanocytes. In: Nathanson L (ed.) *Human Melanoma Research: Genetics, Growth Factors, Metastases, and Antigens*, pp. 19–40. Boston: Kluwer.

Ortonne JP, Mosher DB and Fitzpatrick TB (1982) *Vitiligo and Other Hypomelanoses of Hair and Skin*. New York: Plenum.

Thody AJ (1980) *The MSH Peptides*. London: Academic Press.

Thody AJ and Friedmann PS (eds) (1986) *Scientific Basis of Dermatology: A Physiological Approach*. Edinburgh: Churchill Livingstone.

Yaar M and Gilchrest BA (1991) Human melanocyte growth and differentiation: a decade of new data. *Journal of Investigative Dermatology* **97**, 611–617.

4 The Epidermal Basement Membrane

MICHAEL J. TIDMAN

Basement membranes represent structurally and biochemically distinct parts of the extracellular matrix. There are several basement membranes to be found in human skin, including those around vascular channels and nerves and associated with muscle and fat cells. However, the basement membrane of most interest to dermatologists is that separating the epidermis and dermis, the epidermal basement membrane (EBM). This is a dynamic structure, undergoing constant remodelling, that forms a continuous interface between the epidermis and the dermis (the dermo-epidermal junction) and, as such, it is thought to have a number of essential functions, including the support and attachment of epidermal cells, the regulation of nutritional transport between dermis and epidermis, and the control of epidermal development and organisation. The EBM appears to play an integral part in such physiological and pathological processes as wound healing, the spread of epidermal neoplasms and blistering in a variety of inherited and acquired bullous disorders. Over the last 15 years, the interest in these fundamental processes has stimulated considerable research into the composition of the EBM.

STRUCTURE OF THE EPIDERMAL BASEMENT MEMBRANE

The EBM is beyond the limits of resolution of the light microscope, but at the ultrastructural level the electron microscope shows a fairly complex morphology (Figs 4.1 and 4.2). It has, like other basement membranes, a basic bilamellar structure. The two laminae are named the lamina lucida and the lamina densa, and these structures lie parallel to the irregularly convoluted plasma membrane of the basal epidermal cells, together constituting a virtually uninterrupted sheet between normal epidermis and dermis. The lamina lucida, which separates the lamina densa from the plasma membrane of the basal epidermal cells, appears relatively empty under the electron microscope, apart from numerous slender anchoring filaments which cross it perpendicularly from the basal plasma membrane to the lamina densa. These anchoring filaments, which have no discernible fine structure, are particularly numerous and well ordered in the region of the hemidesmosomes. The electron lucency of the lamina

Molecular Aspects of Dermatology. Edited by G.C. Priestley.
© 1993 by John Wiley & Sons Ltd

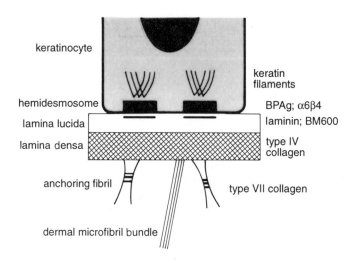

keratinocyte

keratin filaments

hemidesmosome

BPAg; α6β4

lamina lucida

laminin; BM600

lamina densa

type IV collagen

anchoring fibril

type VII collagen

dermal microfibril bundle

Fig. 4.1. Schematic diagram of the epidermal basement membrane showing major structural elements and molecular components

lucida, however, belies its complex chemical constitution. The lamina densa has a natural electron density, which is usually enhanced by routine electron microscopic stains. It has a homogeneous fine granular or fibrillar appearance, and tends to be widest beneath hemidesmosomes.

Hemidesmosomes are complex electron-dense structures, studded at frequent, but irregular, intervals along keratinocyte-associated EBM. They consist of an intracellular portion, the attachment plaque, which lies within the basal keratinocyte on the inner side of the basal plasma membrane, and which has an intimate association with the keratin intermediate filaments (tonofilaments). The sub-basal dense plate of the hemidesmosome is a narrow zone of electron-dense material lying within the lamina lucida, parallel to the attachment plaque, and traversed by the anchoring filaments.

Immediately beneath the lamina densa, within the superficial dermis are three types of fibrillar structure: anchoring fibrils, dermal microfibril bundles (which represent the terminal arborisations of the elastic system), and collagen fibrils, embedded in a ground substance rich in glycosaminoglycans. The anchoring fibrils are curved structures resembling old-fashioned wheat sheaves, composed of a number of individual filaments. At the extremities of the anchoring fibrils, individual filaments fan out and superficially insert into, and radiate within, the lamina densa. The deep ends of the anchoring fibrils splay out into the dermis and may be embedded in 'anchoring plaques' – islands of lamina densa within the superficial dermis – creating a series of loops through which collagen fibrils may weave. In the mid-portions of the anchoring fibrils the individual filaments are closely packed, and impart a characteristic cross-banding with an irregular periodicity.

It has been suggested that there may be a structural and functional

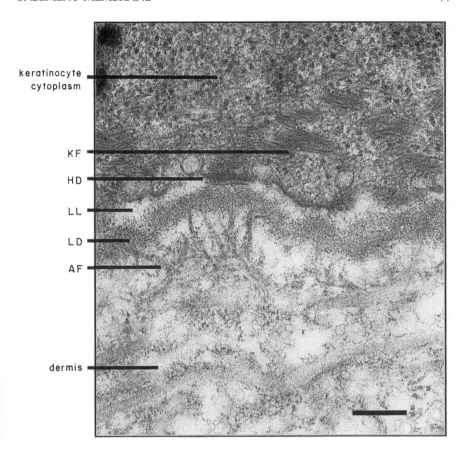

keratinocyte
cytoplasm

KF

HD

LL

LD

AF

dermis

Fig. 4.2. Electron micrograph of the epidermal basement membrane zone. AF, anchoring fibrils; HD, hemidesmosome; KF, keratin filaments; LL, lamina lucida; LD, lamina densa. Calibration bar = 0.25 μm

continuity between the filamentous elements of the sub-lamina densa zone, the anchoring filaments and the intracellular intermediate filaments of basal keratinocytes, and an increasing understanding of the molecular constituents of the EBM and their interaction lends support to this concept.

BIOCHEMICAL COMPOSITION OF THE EPIDERMAL BASEMENT MEMBRANE

It is convenient to consider the chemical composition of the EBM in terms of the ultrastructural regions, although the apparent segregation of macro-molecules between the lamina lucida and the lamina densa may be misleading. The very small amount of EBM in skin samples has hindered its chemical analysis, and most of our knowledge stems either from studies of tumour cell lines producing basement membrane-like material in large quantities, or from the use of characterised antibodies. Using these techniques, it has become apparent that the EBM is composed of a wide variety of glycoproteins and other macromolecules, some of which are shared with other basement membranes and others which are specific to the basement membrane of stratified squamous epithelium.

LAMININ

Laminin is a ubiquitous component of basement membranes throughout the animal kingdom, and is probably the most abundant non-collagenous protein to be found in basement membranes. In the EBM it occurs principally in the lamina lucida although it is probably also present within the lamina densa.

Laminin is a large glycoprotein of approximately 800 kDa, with some heterogeneity of structure, existing in species- and tissue-specific isoforms. There are at least three major isoforms: classical laminin, merosin (M-laminin) and S-laminin. Each is composed of three genetically distinct polypeptide chains, stabilised by disulphide bonds, and rotary shadowing electron microscopy has demonstrated them to be arranged in an asymmetric cruciate shape. Laminin in the EBM is principally of the classical type, with a large subunit (A chain; 400 kDa) and two smaller polypeptides (B_1 and B_2; M_r 200 kDa). In normal human EBM there is also immunoreactive merosin (Sollberg et al., 1992), in which the A chain of classical laminin is substituted by an M chain (B_1–M–B_2). S-Laminin (S–A–B_2) is not present in normal EBM; it is usually to be found in neural tissue, but appears to be expressed around islands of basal cell carcinomas (Sollberg et al., 1992).

Each of the three polypeptides of laminin possess multiple structural domains, and all three chains share considerable homology. Certain domains within all three chains contain amino acid repeats showing close homology to epidermal growth factor (EGF), and these EGF-like domains appear to be highly conserved across the evolutionary spectrum, suggesting that they may have vitally important functions.

The laminin molecule is richly glycosylated at sites which are unevenly distributed over the molecule. The carbohydrate content is principally oligosaccharide, and the significance of glycosylation has yet to be determined, although it may be involved in cell–matrix interactions.

Laminin is able to self-aggregate and this function appears to be calcium dependent. Subsequent enzyme-mediated cross-linking between laminin molecules may serve to stabilise the laminin structure within basement membranes. It is a very biologically active molecule with an affinity for type IV collagen and heparan sulphate proteoglycan and probably thereby plays an important role in maintaining the cohesion of basement membranes. Laminin also promotes cell attachment, probably via an interaction between specific cellular binding sites and the integrin family of cell adhesion receptors

(Gehlson *et al.*, 1988), inhibits keratinocyte migration and promotes keratinocyte proliferation and differentiation.

ENTACTIN/NIDOGEN

Entactin and nidogen were the names given to macromolecules isolated from different sources of basement membrane, which have subsequently been shown to be identical proteins of 150 kDa. Entactin/nidogen is expressed with laminin, and is probably an integral part of the laminin molecule, forming a non-covalent complex in basement membranes. Rotary shadowing electron microscopy has shown entactin/nidogen to have a dumb-bell shaped structure, with one large and one small globule connected by a rod-like domain. It binds by one of its globular domains to one of the short arms of laminin. The rod-like domain contains EGF-like amino acid repeats. Post-translational modifications of entactin/nidogen include glycosylation and tyrosine sulphation. It is thought that the entactin/nidogen molecule may serve to link laminin and type IV collagen molecules.

TYPE IV COLLAGEN

Type IV collagen is the main collagenous element of all basement membranes, and immuno-electron microscopic studies have demonstrated that it is located in the lamina densa and anchoring plaques of the EBM. Each molecule of type IV collagen consists of three polypeptide chains, each approximately 180 kDa. In human type IV collagen there are two types of polypeptide chain, $\alpha1(IV)$ and $\alpha2(IV)$, with each molecule of collagen being composed of two $\alpha1$ chains and one $\alpha2$ chain. An isoform of type IV collagen, containing a recently identified type IV collagen polypeptide chain, $\alpha5$, may be present in normal EBM (Kashtan *et al.*, 1986).

The type IV collagen molecule, consisting of the three polypeptide chains united along most of their length in the form of a triple helix, appears to be composed of three major domains. The 7S domain is present at the N-terminus and is 13 nm in length and rich in cysteine and lysine residues. At the C-terminus there is a non-collagenous NC1 domain, which has a globular structure. Between these two domains is the major part of the triple helix, measuring 360 nm in length and containing frequent interruptions in the typical Gly–X–Y repeat structure of collagen helices.

The collagenous meshwork of the lamina densa of the EBM is formed by the self-assembly of type IV collagen molecules, which are able to cross-link with each other by disulphide bonds. Dimerisation occurs via the interaction of NC1 domains between two molecules, and tetramer formation results from the association of four molecules via their 7S domains. Subsequently, lateral interactions between the triple helices also occur, and these three forms of interaction provide a strong network that serves as a scaffold for the basement membrane.

HEPARAN SULPHATE PROTEOGLYCAN

The proteoglycans found within basement membranes are not yet as well characterised as laminin or type IV collagen. Variations of both the protein core and the glycosaminoglycan component probably account for some diversity in the proteoglycan composition of different basement membranes.

Immunohistochemical studies have shown that heparan sulphate proteoglycan is a widespread constituent of basement membrane, including the dermo-epidermal junction, and it is likely that this macromolecule is the principal proteoglycan. The anionic nature of heparan sulphate proteoglycan makes it a contender for a role in the filtration properties of the EBM. A model of the ultrastructural localisation of the biochemical constituents of the EBM places heparan sulphate proteoglycan on the superficial and deep aspects of the lamina densa, but it seems likely that proteoglycan is incorporated into the type IV collagen meshwork, although the mechanism of interaction with laminin and type IV collagen is unknown.

By analogy with other basement membranes, it seems likely that the heparan sulphate proteoglycan within the EBM is heterogeneous in composition, with different sized protein cores and varying ratios of glycosaminoglycans to protein.

Another proteoglycan relatively recently identified in the EBM contains chondroitin-6-sulphate. Its precise function is unknown, but its immunohistochemical expression is impaired in recessive and dominant forms of dystrophic epidermolysis bullosa (Fine and Couchman, 1988).

BULLOUS PEMPHIGOID ANTIGENS

Bullous pemphigoid is an autoimmune disorder, characterised clinically by the formation of large tense blisters, which develop within the lamina lucida of the dermo-epidermal junction, associated with itchy inflamed skin. It can develop at any time of life, but is most common in the elderly. An auto-antibody of the IgG class is produced, and this is frequently detectable in the circulation and almost always detectable in the skin of affected patients, bound in a linear fashion along the EBM. Although this antibody can bind complement and activate the classical and alternative complement pathways, relatively little is known about the precise mechanisms leading to dermo-epidermal separation, and the evidence that the bullous pemphigoid antibody is directly pathogenic is still rather circumstantial. Nonetheless, its presence has enabled the characterisation of its target antigen, bullous pemphigoid antigen (BP Ag).

Immunogold ultrastructural studies have demonstrated BP Ag to be predominantly intracellular, associated with the attachment plaque of the hemidesmosome, but there is also a small extracellular pool within the lamina lucida. In fact, immunoblotting and immunoprecipitation studies have shown there to be two immunologically distinct target antigens in bullous pemphigoid, and recent molecular genetic studies have shown these two antigens to be the product of different genes on separate chromosomes (Sawamura et al., 1992). The major BP Ag (BP Ag1) has an M_r of 230 kDa and a central coiled-coil α-helical rod structure, and is a constituent of the intracellular hemidesmosomal attachment plaque. It is of interest that it is homologous to the desmosomal protein desmoplakin I, which suggests that it may have a role in dermo-epidermal adhesion. The second BP Ag (BP Ag2) is smaller (180 kDa) and is also found within the attachment plaque of the hemidesmosome. However, its structure suggests that it is a highly conserved transmembrane protein (Guidice et al., 1992; Hopkinson et al., 1992). It has an unusual composition, with a long extracellular collagenous tail, suggesting that it may function as a cell–matrix adhesion molecule. The orientation of the molecule with respect to the plasma membrane is also very unusual for a transmembrane protein, as the carboxy terminus is extracellular and the amino terminus is within the cytoplasm. The extracellular collagenous portion of the molecule consists of a number of collagen-like domains, separated from each other by short non-collagenous segments.

BP Ag2 is the target antigen in another bullous disease, herpes (pemphigoid) gestationis. This is also an autoimmune condition in which an avidly complement-fixing IgG antibody is expressed during the second or third trimester of pregnancy. The result is an intensely itchy blistering eruption that gradually subsides after the pregnancy is completed, often only to recur during subsequent confinements. The epitope identified by the antibody appears to be located in the short non-collagenous extracellular portion of BP Ag2 between the transmembrane and the collagen tail domains.

Yet another bullous disease that appears closely related to bullous pemphigoid is cicatricial pemphigoid. Histologically, immunohistochemically and ultrastructurally, this disease cannot be distinguished from bullous pemphigoid, although clinically it is very distinct with a tendency to involve mucous membranes and to cause the development of scar tissue. Immuno-electron microscopic studies have demonstrated the cicatricial pemphigoid auto-antibody to bind to the lower portion of the lamina lucida and to the lamina densa, beneath hemidesmosomes. Very recent data, however, suggest that the major target antigen in cicatricial pemphigoid is a 180 kDa protein and there is also a 230 kDa minor antigen, and that these two proteins immunologically cross-react with the bullous pemphigoid antigens (Bernard et al., 1992). The reasons for the very different clinical pictures of the two forms of pemphigoid remain to be elucidated.

BM600

BM600 (nicein) is a recently identified constituent of the hemidesmosomes. Its identification came about as the result of the serendipitous production of a monoclonal antibody, GB3, from an amnion immunogen. GB3 proved to recognise an epitope within the EBM, and ultrastructural studies have suggested that it is associated with hemidesmosomes. The recognition that GB3 expression is abnormal in the junctional form of epidermolysis bullosa (Verrando et al., 1991) has prompted further interest in this antibody.

Junctional epidermolysis bullosa is a rare mechano-bullous disorder, inherited in an autosomal recessive manner, and sufferers of this condition blister in response to very minor trauma. The condition is usually lethal within 2 years of birth. The tragedy of such children has occasionally received the journalistic description of 'babies that cannot be cuddled'. It has been well established that a basic defect in junctional epidermolysis bullosa is, in the majority of cases, the formation of morphologically abnormal hemidesmo-somes, and blisters arise by cleavage within the lamina lucida of the dermo-epidermal junction. The aberrant expression of GB3 in junctional epidermolysis bullosa suggests that the epitope recognised by this antibody plays an important function in dermo-epidermal adhesion. Characterisation of GB3 has led to the isolation of BM600 (nicein), which is probably identical or closely related to two other recently described constituents of the EBM: kalinin and epiligrin.

BM600 consists of three disulphide-linked glycoprotein subunits of 100, 125 and 150 kDa. Immuno-electron microscopic localisation of BM600 suggests that it is located principally in that part of the lamina lucida immediately beneath the sub-basal dense plate of the hemidesmosome and it may be a constituent of anchoring filaments.

Sequencing of the cDNA corresponding to two of the BM600 subunits has revealed a certain relationship with human laminin (Verrando et al., 1992). Regions of the 100 kDa subunit show a strong homology with the EGF-like domains of the B2 laminin chain, and the 150 kDa subunit has similar amino acid sequences to the A chain of laminin.

TYPE VII COLLAGEN

Type VII collagen is the major constituent of anchoring fibrils and, although present in only minute amounts in human skin, appears to be a very important molecule for maintaining the integrity of the dermo-epidermal junction.

The clinical significance of anchoring fibrils is that there are morphological and quantitative abnormalities of these structures in the dystrophic form of epidermolysis bullosa. Dystrophic epidermolysis bullosa is a group of inherited disorders characterised by trauma-induced blisters which heal with scarring and milium formation. The condition may be inherited in either an autosomal dominant or an autosomal recessive manner. The dominant form tends to be milder, with blistering occurring over acral bony prominences and with associated nail dystrophy. It is compatible with normal life expectancy and a normal reproductive potential. The localised form of recessive dystrophic epidermolysis bullosa is clinically very similar to the dominant type, whereas the generalised form is a more widespread aggressively scarring disorder, affecting the entire integument, oesophagus, anal canal, the oral cavity and teeth, and occasionally external eye and ear. Severely affected individuals are frequently anaemic, and are predisposed to the development of squamous cell carcinoma at the site of repeated blistering. This latter complication appears to be a major cause of death.

In dominant dystrophic epidermolysis bullosa, anchoring fibrils are significantly reduced in number, but appear morphologically normal, whereas in the severe recessive form normal anchoring fibrils appear to be absent. The cleavage plane in dystrophic epidermolysis bullosa is immediately beneath the lamina densa of the dermo-epidermal junction, the site normally occupied by anchoring fibrils, strongly suggesting that blisters form as a result of the paucity or absence of these structures. Furthermore, the immunohistochemical and immuno-electron microscopic expression of type VII collagen is impaired in dystrophic forms of epidermolysis bullosa to a variable degree, being relatively normal in localised forms and virtually non-existent in the severe recessive variant.

Another clinical condition in which anchoring fibrils appear to play a part is epidermolysis bullosa acquisita, an auto-immune bullous disorder characterised by chronic blistering. The clinical features of this condition are rather variable, and it may mimic such diverse diseases as bullous pemphigoid, cicatricial pemphigoid, dystrophic epidermolysis bullosa and porphyria cutanea tarda. Epidermolysis bullosa acquisita is characterised by the deposition of immuno-globulins, usually IgG, at the dermo-epidermal junction with the cleavage plane beneath the lamina densa. Approximately 50% of patients with epidermolysis bullosa acquisita have circulating antibodies against type VII collagen.

Type VII collagen is synthesised by both keratinocytes and dermal fibroblasts, and is the largest member of the collagen family, with the triple helical portion measuring approximately 450 nm. Each molecule is composed of three identical α chains, $\alpha1(VII)$, and each α chain is synthesised as a procollagen, pro-$\alpha1(VII)$. The procollagen molecule has a molecular weight of approximately 300–350 kDa, and consists of a central rod-like collagenous domain of approximately 145 kDa, a large globular non-collagenous domain (NC1) at the amino terminal with a molecular weight of approximately 145 kDa, and a much smaller non-collagenous domain (NC2), of approximately 30 kDa, at the carboxyl end of the molecule. The collagenous domain of type VII collagen contains a number of non-collagenous segments, and it appears that these interruptions within the triple helix serve to increase the flexibility of the molecule. In addition, the large NC1 domain also contains subdomains including several segments with homology to fibronectin, to which type VII collagen has a specific affinity. These sequences within the NC1 domain may therefore play an important part in the attachment function of the anchoring fibrils.

The first step in the assembly of anchoring fibrils in the extracellular space is the formation of anti-parallel dimers. Two procollagen molecules align themselves end-to-end at their carboxy termini, and they are then linked and stabilised by disulphide bonds, following which the NC2 domains are proteolytically cleaved. The second step is the lateral aggregation of a large number of these dimer molecules. It is thought that the large NC1 domain interacts with type IV collagen, laminin and fibonectin within the lamina densa superficially and the anchoring plaques more deeply, thereby contributing to dermo-epidermal adhesion.

The gene coding for type VII collagen, COL7A1, has recently been localised to the short arm of chromosome 3, and genetic linkage studies strongly suggest that both the dominant and the recessive forms of dystrophic epidermolysis bullosa are the result of mutations in the COL7A1 gene. The precise nature of these mutations should be defined in the very near future. It seems likely that a spectrum of mutations will account for the variety of clinical manifestations of dystrophic epidermolysis bullosa.

INTEGRINS

Integrins are cell surface glycoprotein heterodimers that consist of two different chains (α and β) that are linked in a non-covalent fashion. Their importance is that they function as receptors in cell–cell and cell–matrix interactions. Integrin receptors associate with extracellular ligands, and fibronectin, laminin and type IV collagen are known to be ligands for different integrins, suggesting that integrins may play an important role in the structural and functional integrity of the EBM. There is convincing evidence for a role for integrins in mediating cell attachment to laminin and type IV collagen. Furthermore, the cytoplasmic domains of a number of integrin receptors have an indirect connection with the actin – and perhaps the intermediate filament – cytoskeleton, providing a possible biochemical pathway across the cell membrane between intracellular structural proteins and extracellular matrix proteins, such as laminin, types IV and VII collagen and fibronectin. Thus, integrin receptors may act as signal transducers through which extracellular matrix proteins can activate and modify cellular functions, and it also appears likely that, via integrin receptors, cells can modify the nature of their extracellular environment.

The integrin family is divided into subfamilies on the basis of the β subunits, and there are at least six different β chains. Both α and β chains have a cytoplasmic domain (carboxy terminal), which is usually quite short, a transmembrane domain and a large globular extracellular domain (amino terminal). Binding of the integrin to its ligand requires both the α and β subunits and depends not only on the presence of divalent cations but also on specific amino acid sequences in the ligand, of which the arginine–glycine–aspartic acid (RGD) sequence is perhaps the most common. However, by no means all integrin–ligand interactions occur via this peptide. Some integrins interact with specific ligands, such as laminin or fibronectin, while others are able to bind to multiple ligands. The molecular basis for the recognition mechanisms between integrins and their ligands is unclear.

Integrin α6β4 is expressed on the lower pole of basal keratinocytes and is localised to the hemidesmosomes (Carter et al., 1990; Stepp et al., 1990; Sonnenberg et al., 1991). It is considered to have a role in adhesion of the basal cells to the EBM. The β4 chain, unlike the majority of integrin subunits, has a comparatively large cytoplasmic domain which appears to be an important component of the hemidesmosome attachment plaque. The ligand of α6β4 remains to be determined, but it may prove to be laminin or perhaps BM600. There is speculation that a defect of the α6β4 integrin may be involved in the pathogenesis of subepidermal blistering disorders, although no abnormality of integrin expression has yet been found in the inherited forms of epidermolysis bullosa (Nazzaro et al., 1990).

At least two other integrins, α2β1 and α3β1, are also expressed at the EBM (Eberhard Klein et al., 1990). Both are laminin-binding integrins and α2β1 also binds to type IV collagen, and the α3β1 receptor has an affinity for epiligrin (Carter et al., 1991). It therefore seems likely that these two integrins are also involved in the adhesion of keratinocytes to the EBM.

MISCELLANEOUS

The complement component C3d,g has been detected in the EBM (Basset-Seguin et al., 1988) and the presence of complement components may be the means for the fixation of immune complexes and the initiation of the inflammatory processes in the immunological disorders that involve the EBM zone.

Biologically active basic fibroblast growth factor has been demonstrated to be bound to, and perhaps stored in, basement membranes (Folkman et al., 1988). This growth factor has an affinity for the heparan sulphate proteoglycan. Other growth factors may also be present within basement membranes.

Several different protein moieties are thought to contribute to the delicate wisp-like microfilamentous structures visible by transmission electron microscopy in the sub-lamina densa fibrous zone. As well as type VII collagen, type VI collagen (Keene et al., 1988) and two non-collagenous proteins, linkin (Yoshiike et al., 1988) and fibrillin (Sakai et al., 1986), may contribute to the wispy arrangement beneath the lamina densa. Fibrillin is a globular glycoprotein (350 kDa) which forms the microfibrillar scaffold of the elastic fibres. A mutation in the gene for fibrillin is responsible for Marfan's syndrome. Linkin consists of two microfilament proteins (73 and 83 kDa), which span the spaces between anchoring fibrils and elastic microfibrils, and are considered to assist in holding connective tissue components together.

There are several basement membrane-associated glycoproteins, including thrombospondin, tenascin and SPARC (secreted protein acidic and rich in cysteine), that appear to have repulsive properties and may function to modulate the adhesive effects of laminin and fibronectin. These proteins are not confined to basement membranes, although there is a Ca^{2+}-dependent binding of SPARC to type IV collagen (Mayer et al., 1991). They may influence the behaviour of connective tissue cells such as fibroblasts, smooth muscle cells and endothelial cells.

A further number of EBM antigens, which have not yet been fully characterised, have been identified on the basis of their reactivity with monoclonal antibodies. The antibody LDA-1 recognises a basement membrane epitope, composed of two low-molecular-weight proteins (45 and 51.5 kDa), that has a wide tissue distribution, including the EBM, and is localised to the lamina densa (Fine and Gay, 1986). The antibody 19-DEJ-1 identifies a hemidesmosome-associated epitope present within the lamina lucida, perhaps as part of the anchoring filaments. The interest in 19-DEJ-1 is that its expression is absent in all patients with junctional epidermolysis bullosa and in some patients with recessive dystrophic epidermolysis bullosa (Fine et al., 1989). Recently NUT 2, a mouse monoclonal antibody recognising the CD1b molecule expressed by cortical thymocytes and some dendritic cells, has been demonstrated to recognise an epitope within the lower part of the lamina lucida of the EBM. The NUT 2 antigen has still to be characterised and it remains to be determined whether it has a function in the transfer of immunocompetent cells across the EBM (Kanitakis et al., 1992).

Finally, the blistering disorder linear IgA disease is characterised by the deposition of IgA in a linear fashion along the EBM. However, it appears to be a heterogeneous disorder with the antibody localising to the lamina lucida or the sub-lamina densa zone. Presumably, this variation reflects different target antigens.

CONCLUSIONS

The EBM seems to be a veritable soup of interacting protein molecules, some ubiquitous to all basement membranes and others present only at the dermo-epidermal junction. Focal and regional variations within the EBM, for instance around appendageal structures and beneath melanocytes, may reflect functional differences at these sites. Knowledge of the molecular composition of basement membranes is expanding rapidly, and a more complete understanding of the biochemical nature of the EBM will almost certainly pave the way for major advances in the fields of wound healing, metastatic spread of epidermal neoplasms and acquired and inherited blistering disorders.

REFERENCES

Basset-Seguin N, Dersookian M, Cehrs K and Yancey KB (1988) C3d,g is present in normal human epidermal basement membrane. *Journal of Immunology* **141**, 1273–1280.

Bernard P, Prost C, Durepaire N, Basset-Seguin N, Didierjean L and Saurat J-H (1992) The major cicatricial pemphigoid antigen is a 180kD protein that shows immunologic cross-reactivities with the bullous pemphigoid antigen. *Journal of Investigative Dermatology* **99**, 174–179.

Carter WG, Kaur P, Gill SG, Gahr PJ and Wayner EA (1990) Distinct functions for integrins $\alpha 3\beta 1$ in focal adhesions and $\alpha 6\beta 4$/bullous pemphigoid antigen in a new stable anchoring contact (SAC) of keratinocytes: relation to hemidesmosomes. *Journal of Cell Biology* **111**, 3141–3154.

Carter WG, Ryan MC and Gahr PJ (1991) Epiligrin, a new cell adhesion ligand for integrin $\alpha 3\beta 1$ in epithelial basement membranes. *Cell* **65**, 599–610.

Eberhard Klein C, Steinmayer T, Mattes JM, Kaufmann R and Weber L (1990) Integrins of normal human epidermis: differential expression, synthesis and molecular structure. *British Journal of Dermatology* **123**, 171–178.

Fine JD and Couchman JR (1988) Chondroitin-6-sulfate-containing proteoglycan: a new component of human skin dermo-epidermal junction. *Journal of Investigative Dermatology* **90**, 283–288.

Fine JD and Gay S (1986) Characterization of a new ubiquitous non-collagenous component of basement membrane as defined by monoclonal antibody technique. *Journal of Investigative Dermatology* **86**, 475 (abstract).

Fine JD, Hariguchi Y and Couchman JR (1989) 19-DEJ-1, a hemidesmosome-anchoring filament complex-associated monoclonal antibody. Definition of a new skin basement membrane antigenic defect in junctional and dystrophic epidermolysis bullosa. *Archives of Dermatology* **125**, 520–523.

Folkman J, Klagsbrun M, Sasse J, Wadzinski M, Ingber D and Vlodavsky I (1988) A heparin-binding angiogenic protein, a basic fibroblast growth factor, is stored within basement membrane. *American Journal of Pathology* **130**, 393–400.

Gehlsen KR, Dillner L, Engvall E and Ruoslahti E (1988) The human laminin receptor is a member of the integrin family of cell adhesion receptors. *Science* **241**, 1228–1229.

Guidice GJ, Emery DJ and Diaz LA (1992) Cloning and primary structural analysis of the bullous pemphigoid autoantigen BP180. *Journal of Investigative Dermatology* **99**, 243–250.

Hopkinson SB, Riddelle KS and Jones JCR (1992) Cytoplasmic domain of the 180kD bullous pemphigoid antigen, a hemidesmosomal component: molecular and cell biologic characterization. *Journal of Investigative Dermatology* **99**, 264–270.

Kanitakis J, Wang YZ, Zambruno G and Schmitt D (1992) Reactivity of an anti-CD1b monoclonal antibody (NUT2) with a (novel?) antigen of the dermal–epidermal junction. *Clinical and Experimental Dermatology* **17**, 294 (abstract).

Kashtan C, Fish AJ, Kleppel M, Yoshioka K and Michael AF (1986) Nephritogenic antigen determinants in epidermal and renal basement membranes of kindreds with Alport-type familial nephritis. *Journal of Clinical Investigation* **78**, 1035–1044.

Keene DR, Engvall E and Glanville RW (1988) Ultrastructure of type VI collagen in human skin and cartilage suggests an anchoring function for this filamentous network. *Journal of Cell Biology* **107**, 1995–2006.

Mayer U, Aumailley M, Mann K, Timpl R and Engel J (1991) Calcium-dependent binding of basement protein BM-40 (osteonectin, SPARC) to basement membrane collagen type IV. *European Journal of Biochemistry* **198**, 141–150.

Nazzaro V, Berti E, Cerri A, Brusasco A, Cavalli R and Caputo R (1990) Expression of integrins in junctional and dystrophic epidermolysis bullosa. *Journal of Investigative Dermatology* **95**, 60–64.

Sakai LY, Keene DR and Engvall E (1986) Fibrillin, a new 350 kD glycoprotein, is a component of extracellular microfibrils. *Journal of Cell Biology* **103**, 2499–2506.

Sawamura D, Li K and Uitto J (1992) 230kD and 180kD bullous pemphigoid antigens are distinct gene products. *Journal of Investigative Dermatology* **98**, 942–943.

Sollberg S, Peltonen J and Uitto J (1992) Differential expression of laminin isoforms and β4 integrin epitopes in the basement membrane zone of normal human skin and basal cell carcinomas. *Journal of Investigative Dermatology* **98**, 864–870.

Sonnenberg A, Calafat J, Janssen H, Daams H, van der Raaij-Helmer LMH, Falcioni R, Kennel SJ, Aplin JD, Baker J, Loizidou M and Garrod D (1991) Integrin a6β4 complex is located in hemidesmosomes, suggesting a major role in epidermal cell–basement membrane adhesion. *Journal of Cell Biology* **113**, 907–917.

Stepp MA, Spurr-Michaud S, Tisdale A, Elwell J and Gipson IK (1990) α6β4 integrin heterodimer is a component of hemidesmosomes. *Proceedings of the National Academy of Sciences USA* **87**, 8970–8974.

Verrando P, Blanchet-Bardon C, Pisani A, Thomas L, Cambazard F, Eady RAJ, Schofield O and Ortonne JP (1991) Monoclonal antibody GB3 defines a widespread defect of several basement membranes and a keratinocyte dysfunction in patients with lethal junctional epidermolysis bullosa. *Laboratory Investigation* **64**, 85–92.

Verrando P, Vailly J, Baudoin C, Meneguzzi G and Ortonne JP (1992) Molecular cloning and sequence of cDNAs coding for a subunit of the basement membrane protein BM600 (niceine). *Journal of Investigative Dermatology* **98**, 824 (abstract).

Yoshiike T, Briggaman RA, Woodley DT, Gammon WR and Cronce DJ (1988) Identification and partial characterisation of a microthread-like filamentous network beneath human skin basement membrane zone. *Journal of Investigative Dermatology* **90** 620 (abstract).

SUGGESTIONS FOR FURTHER READING

Eady RAJ (1988) The basement membrane. Interface between the epithelium and the dermis: structural features. *Archives of Dermatology* **124**, 709–712.

Fine J-D (1988) Antigenic features and structural correlates of basement membranes: relationship to epidermolysis bullosa. *Archives of Dermatology* **124**, 713–717.

Paulsson M (1992) Basement membrane proteins: structure, assembly and cellular interactions. *Critical Reviews in Biochemistry and Molecular Biology* **27**, 93–127.

Uitto J, Chung-Honet LC and Christiano AM (1992) Molecular biology and pathology of type VII collagen. *Experimental Dermatology* **1**, 2–11.

5 Proteoglycans and Glycosaminoglycans

MICHAEL EDWARD

The dermis has a basic structure like that of other connective tissues, a composite system of insoluble fibrils and soluble polymers which take the stresses of movement and maintain shape. The insoluble fibres are collagen and elastin, while the major soluble macromolecules are proteoglycans and hyaluronan, which bind vast amounts of water, and thus occupy a large volume. The fibrous components of skin resist tensile forces, while the proteoglycans and hyaluronan resist or dissipate compressive forces. Proteoglycans were previously considered to be inert structural components of connective tissues, where they are present in relatively high concentrations and they determine the physical properties of the tissue. However, we are now aware that this complex and diverse family of macromolecules are synthesised by all types of mammalian cells, and help to regulate cellular growth, adhesion, migration and differentiation. Recently, proteoglycans have also been implicated in regulating the activities of certain growth factors. In view of these properties, proteoglycans and hyaluronan will undoubtedly play vital parts in wound healing and are likely to be involved in the pathogenesis of several dermatological disorders, which will be discussed in this chapter.

STRUCTURE OF GLYCOSAMINOGLYCANS

Glycosaminoglycans are linear polysaccharides in which the inherent structural feature is a repeating disaccharide unit composed of a uronic acid and a hexosamine. The exception to this is keratan sulphate, in which the repeating disaccharide is galactose and N-acetylglucosamine; however, as this glycosaminoglycan has been identified in only small amounts in the epidermis, it will not be discussed further. Hyaluronic acid is the simplest of the glycosaminoglycans, being synthesised as a free polysaccharide chain not linked to a protein or polypeptide; it is non-sulphated, and is composed of a repeating disaccharide of N-acetylglucosamine and glucuronic acid. Hyaluronate is synthesised at the inner side of the plasma membrane by alternate transfer

Molecular Aspects of Dermatology. Edited by G.C. Priestley.
© 1993 by John Wiley & Sons Ltd

of UDP–N-acetylglucosamine and UDP–glucuronic acid to the reducing end of the growing polysaccharide chain which extrudes directly to the exterior. The molecular weight of hyaluronate is normally high, often as great as 7000 kDa, and the molecules exist as open random coil structures which occupy large solvent domains and produce highly viscous solutions. An increased deposition of hyaluronate has been correlated with the onset of cellular migration during several stages of embryonic development and wound healing, and with cellular proliferation. Hyaluronate forms supramolecular structures with certain proteoglycans, the most frequently studied being the large cartilage proteoglycan, aggrecan, such composite structures contributing to the properties of the matrices in which they occur. However, dermal fibroblasts synthesise a large chondroitin sulphate proteoglycan, versican, that also possesses a hyaluronate-binding domain in its core protein. Hyaluronate also binds to specific cell surface receptors, members of the CD44 group of receptors.

Unlike hyaluronate, the sulphated glycosaminoglycans are synthesised by membrane-bound enzymes in the Golgi system which polymerise monosaccharide precursors onto protein acceptors. The linkage region consists of xylose–galactose–galactose–uronic acid, in which the xylose is linked to a serine residue in the protein core, and the first uronic acid is followed by the repeating disaccharide unit. The sulphated glycosaminoglycans can be divided into two major groups: the chondroitin and dermatan sulphates, and the heparin and heparan sulphates. Chondroitin sulphate is composed of a repeating disaccharide of N-acetylgalactosamine and glucuronic acid, which is then subjected to polymer modification, which may include sulphation of either carbons 4 or 6 of the galactosamine unit. Dermatan sulphate contains the same repeat unit as chondroitin sulphate, but in addition a variable number of the glucuronic acid residues, normally linked to the 4-sulphated isomer of N-acetylgalactosamine, are epimerised at carbon 5 to form iduronic acid, which may then be sulphated at carbon 2. The chondroitin and dermatan sulphates often consist of mixed isomers, where chondroitins may contain both 4- and 6-sulphated galactosamine residues, while dermatan sulphate is invariably a copolymer of iduronate- and glucuronate-containing disaccharide units.

Heparin and heparan sulphate are composed of a repeating disaccharide unit of N-acetylglucosamine and glucuronic acid, and like the chondroitins are subjected to polymer modifications. The modifications include N-deacetylation and N-sulphation of the N-acetylglucosamine unit, carbon 5 epimerisation of glucuronic acid, and O-sulphation at carbon 6 of glucosamine residues. In addition, O-sulphate substitutions are infrequently found at carbon 3 of glucosamine units and at carbon 2 of the glucuronic acid units. Overall, the polymer modifications in heparin and heparan sulphate are more extensive than those of the chondroitins and, as many are incomplete, a highly diverse range of macromolecules exists. The basic sugar constituents of the glycosaminoglycans are shown in Fig. 5.1. The distinction between heparin

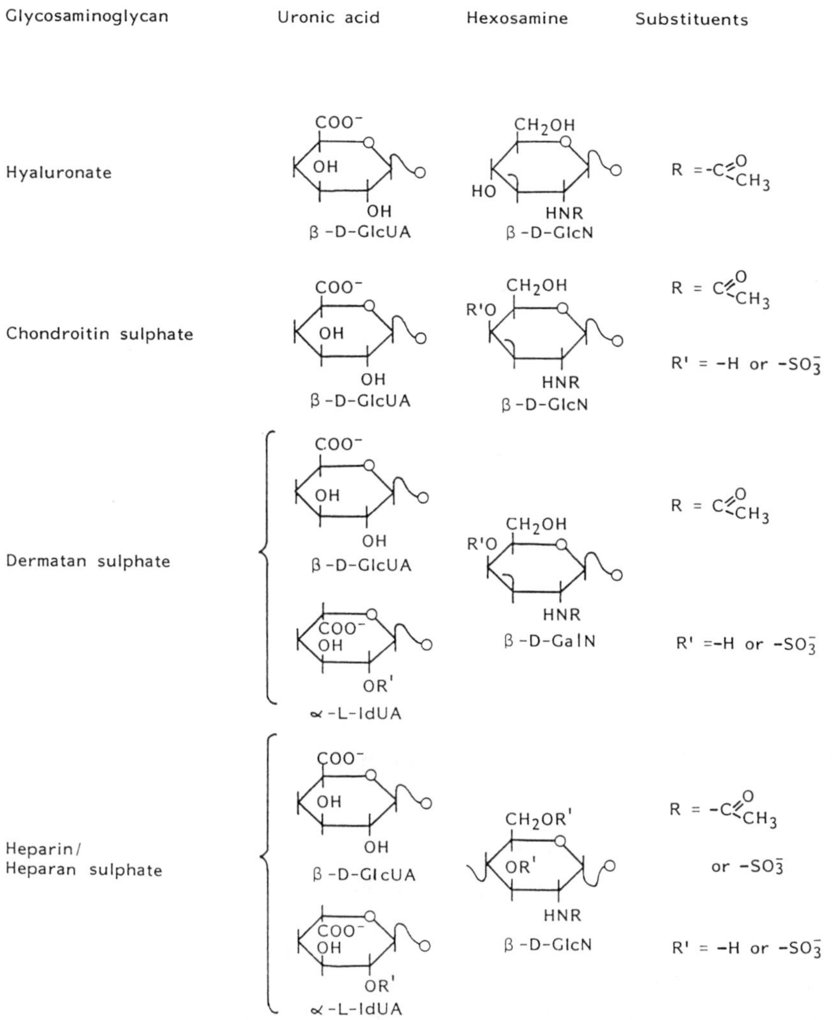

Glycosaminoglycan	Uronic acid	Hexosamine	Substituents
Hyaluronate	COO^- OH OH β-D-GlcUA	CH_2OH HO HNR β-D-GlcN	$R = -C{\overset{O}{\underset{CH_3}{}}}$
Chondroitin sulphate	COO^- OH OH β-D-GlcUA	CH_2OH R'O HNR β-D-GlcN	$R = C{\overset{O}{\underset{CH_3}{}}}$ $R' = -H$ or $-SO_3^-$
Dermatan sulphate	COO^- OH OH β-D-GlcUA COO^- OH OR' α-L-IdUA	CH_2OH R'O HNR β-D-GalN	$R = C{\overset{O}{\underset{CH_3}{}}}$ $R' = -H$ or $-SO_3^-$
Heparin/ Heparan sulphate	COO^- OH OH β-D-GlcUA COO^- OH OR' α-L-IdUA	CH_2OR' OR' HNR β-D-GlcN	$R = -C{\overset{O}{\underset{CH_3}{}}}$ or $-SO_3^-$ $R' = -H$ or $-SO_3^-$

Fig. 5.1. Structure of glycosaminoglycans

and heparan sulphate is not as clear-cut as that between chondroitin sulphate and dermatan sulphate, where dermatan sulphate is characterised by containing iduronic acid. However, in general heparan sulphate contains fewer N- and O-sulphate groups and iduronic acid units than heparin, and more N-acetylglucosamine and glucuronic acid residues. In addition, the various modifications and substitutions are not evenly distributed along the polymer chain. In heparan sulphate, disaccharide units such as N-acetylglucosamine and glucuronic acid appear to co-distribute preferentially, forming block structures interspersed between N-sulphated, more extensively modified sequences. In addition, isolated N-acetylglucosamine residues surrounded by N-sulphated glucosamine residues are commonly found in heparin, while N-sulphated glucosamine units interrupting extended N-acetylated block structures or alternating with N-acetylated disaccharide units are typical of heparan sulphate.

Many interactions of glycosaminoglycans with other molecules are charge-related, and non-specific. Indeed the highly sulphated dextran sulphate can bind to many ligands, such as fibronectin, as avidly as heparin. However, such interactions do not necessarily imply a biological function, and under physiological conditions it is heparan sulphate rather than heparin that is likely to be involved in protein interactions. The extensive variability in the arrangement of the component sugars within the glycosaminoglycan chains will undoubtedly result in diverse interactions, with some arrangements conferring highly specific properties upon the polymer chain. For example, the 3-O-sulphated, N-sulphated glucosamine residue is an essential component of a pentasaccharide sequence in heparin that is responsible for its binding to antithrombin III and for potent anticoagulant activity, and which may also be present in heparan sulphate proteoglycan produced by endothelial cells. Structural differences may also be important in heparan sulphate in regulating cellular growth, as heparans isolated from normal rat liver inhibit the growth of hepatoma cells, while heparans produced by confluent smooth muscle cells inhibit the growth of subconfluent cells.

STRUCTURE OF PROTEOGLYCANS

Proteoglycans are amazingly complex macromolecules composed of a protein core to which is covalently bound one or more sulphated glycosaminoglycan chains. The great structural diversity of the chains provides a wide variety of biological functions. Many protein cores have now been identified, but in general they lack distinctive features that would enable them to be classified into a particular group, or even to predict whether they would carry a glycosaminoglycan chain. The protein core may function as a simple scaffold for immobilisation and spacing of glycosaminoglycan chains; however, the sequence data obtained from recombinant DNA techniques have revealed that many core proteins contain functional domains that may be ascribed to, for example, integration into the plasma membrane or interaction with other extracellular matrix macromolecules.

The proteoglycans may be intracellular, extracellular, or part of a pericellular envelope. The cell-associated proteoglycans may be attached to the cell in several different ways. Those which are integral components of the plasma membrane typically have a hydrophobic core protein domain which is intercalated in the lipid bilayer. Such proteoglycans usually possess an intracellular domain which interacts with the cytoskeleton, while the extracellular protein domain, together with its attached glycosaminoglycan chains, is

Table 5.1. Proteoglycans (PG) of skin

Epidermis	Heparan sulphate PG, keratan sulphate PG, chondroitin sulphate PG, PG-100, CD44, syndecan
Basement membrane	Heparan sulphate PG, chondroitin sulphate PG
Dermis	Heparan sulphate PG, chondroitin sulphate PG, dermatan sulphate PG, decorin, biglycan, fibroglycan, versican, glypican

free to interact with other extracellular matrix molecules. One such proteo-glycan, recently identified, is syndecan, which appears to be associated with epithelial cell membranes. Different cells produce various syndecan molecules differing in the size, number, and proportions of heparan sulphate and chondroitin/dermatan sulphate chains. Syndecan from simple epithelia appears to be localised at the basolateral surface, whereas that from stratified epithelia is found all over the cell surface. Some core proteins may be bound to the cell surface through linkage to phosphatidylinositol, while others interact with cell surface receptors. Proteoglycans may also interact with cell surface molecules via their glycosaminoglycan chains, and indeed certain free glycosaminoglycans may also interact, such as hyaluronate with the CD44 receptor. The distribution of several proteoglycans in skin is shown in Table 5.1

The intracellular proteoglycans are normally small, and associated with granules, such as heparin proteoglycan in mast cells. Such proteoglycans usually have a core protein which contains a number of serine–glycine repeats, hence the name serglycin. These repeats determine the location of the glycosaminoglycan side chains which may be either over-sulphated chondroitin sulphates or heparin. In many cases, the chondroitin sulphate chains are found in the serglycin proteoglycans of mucosal mast cells and platelets, while connective tissue mast cells synthesise heparin chains on the core protein, clustering up to 15 chains of approximately 100 kDa in the repeating serine–glycine region.

The extracellular proteoglycans are a heterogeneous group. They vary in size from the small proteoglycan decorin, with a single dermatan sulphate chain, to the multichain chondroitin sulphate proteoglycan versican. Heparan sulphates are the predominant proteoglycans of basement membranes. The variety of proteoglycan structures is shown in Fig. 5.2, and Table 5.2 summarises their properties and possible functions. Decorin, so named because it binds to collagen and when stained appears to 'decorate' the collagen fibres, is characterised by a motif of leucine-rich repeat sequences. It usually contains one chondroitin/dermatan sulphate chain, while a related small proteoglycan, biglycan, contains two such chains. In skin, the chains tend to be predominantly dermatan sulphate with a high percentage of the glucuronic acid residues epimerised to iduronate.

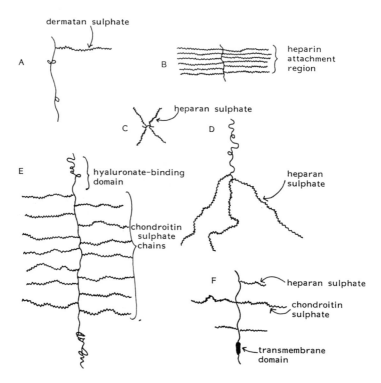

Fig. 5.2. Schematic representation of some putative skin proteoglycans. A: decorin; B: mast cell heparin proteoglycan; C: small basement membrane heparan sulphate proteoglycan; D: large basement membrane heparan sulphate proteoglycan; E: versican; F: syndecan

THE EPIDERMIS

Glycosaminoglycans and proteoglycans in the skin have traditionally been assumed to be synthesised mainly by dermal fibroblasts. However, it is now known that proteoglycans and glycosaminoglycans play vital roles in the epidermis and basement membranes. Metabolic studies utilising both cell and organ culture, and various staining techniques, both in organ culture and *in vivo*, have revealed the presence of both hyaluronate and sulphated glycosaminoglycans in the epidermis. Hyaluronate is the major epidermal glycosaminoglycan, with sulphated glycosaminoglycans (mainly heparan sulphate) as a minor component. Hyaluronate is synthesised by keratinocytes both in cell and organ culture. Undifferentiated, actively proliferating keratinocyte cultures synthesise substantially more hyaluronate than those induced to differentiate, while in addition the presence of the dermal component appears to enhance hyaluronate synthesis by keratinocytes. There is a rapid establishment of cell surface hyaluronate between newly divided keratinocytes, although hyaluronate is not restricted to this zone of

Table 5.2. Structure of some putative skin proteoglycans

Proteoglycan	GAG chains	Core protein size (kDa)	Possible functions
Versican	12–15 CS	265 ⎫	ECM assembly, mechanical
Syndecan	up to 3 HS, 2 CS	32 ⎬	support, cell–cell, cell–matrix interactions, growth factor binding
PG-100	1 C6S	78	Cell adhesion
Biglycan	2 CS/DS	38	Regulation of cell growth and differentiation
Decorin	1 CS/DS	36	Extracellular TGFβ binding, collagen fibrillogenesis
Fibroglycan	HS	48	Cell–cell, cell–matrix interactions, growth factor binding
Glypican	HS	64	Cell–cell, cell–matrix interactions
Serglycin	CS/DS, HS	17–19	Storage and modulation of proteases and protease inhibitors
CD44E	HS/CS	37	Mediate cell adhesion, HA binding
BM HSPGs	4 HS 3 HS	100–130 > 400	Selective filter, growth factor binding, BM assembly

proliferative cells, and appears to predominate in the uppermost spinous cell layer. The levels of hyaluronate in the epidermis, and changes associated with growth and differentiation are consistent with the observations in other cell cultures and tissues that much more hyaluronate is synthesised by proliferating and migrating cells than by stationary differentiated cells.

Treatment of epidermis in organ culture with retinoic acid retards differentiation and stimulates hyaluronate synthesis. In the upper spinous layers increased deposition of hyaluronate may account for the delay in terminal differentiation and weaker cohesion of the keratinocytes (Tammi et al., 1989). This effect of retinoic acid appears to be relatively specific for glycosaminoglycans, as the incorporation of [^{3}H]glucosamine into cultured keratinocytes is increased two- to threefold, while incorporation into glycoproteins remains essentially unaltered. Hyaluronate synthesis decreases as keratinocytes differentiate, but proteoglycan synthesis increases, keeping the same proportions of heparan sulphate and chondroitin sulphate.

Keratinocytes have recently been shown to express CD44 integral membrane glycoproteins and proteoglycans (Brown et al., 1991). The function of CD44 has yet to be determined, although it has been linked with lymphocyte homing and T-cell activation, but its apparently widespread distribution suggests a more general function. This may be as an adhesive cell surface molecule linking extracellular matrix proteins such as collagen, or hyaluronate, with the cytoskeleton. Keratinocytes express particularly high quantities of CD44E in a form termed HS/CS250, which has been identified as a membrane heparan sulphate/chondroitin sulphate proteoglycan and is localised in filopodia and intercellular contacts. Glycosylation of CD44 may be specific for each cell type, with heparan sulphate as the predominant carbohydrate in keratinocytes. The CD44 molecule appears to be distinct from syndecan, however, as the core proteins of the two molecules are unrelated.

BASEMENT MEMBRANES

Proteoglycans are widely distributed in basement membranes, although some forms have a restricted distribution. One of the best-characterised and ubiquitous basement membrane proteoglycans is a large, low buoyant density heparan sulphate proteoglycan, which has a large multidomain protein core greater than 400 kDa, composed of six globular regions of varying sizes. The proteoglycan contains approximately 30% carbohydrate, present as three heparan sulphate chains attached to the protein core at one end. This proteoglycan occurs primarily in the lamina densa and sub-lamina densa region of the dermo-epidermal junction. A second heparan sulphate proteoglycan is found in basement membranes, being of high density, and possessing a small protein core of approximately 100–130 kDa to which are attached four heparan sulphate chains. A chondroitin-6-sulphate proteoglycan has also been identified associated with basement membranes. The highly polyanionic nature of these macromolecules will undoubtedly give them the ability to act as selective filters within the basement membrane, but in addition they may be involved in the assembly and maintenance of basement membranes. Heparan sulphates bind to several extracellular matrix components, including type IV collagen and laminin, which possesses a specific heparin-binding domain. Such interactions have been demonstrated by the formation of basement membrane-like structures *in vitro* following incubation of a mixture of laminin, type IV collagen and heparan sulphate proteoglycan, which had been isolated from the basement membrane-producing EHS tumour.

THE DERMIS

The major glycosaminoglycans of the dermis are hyaluronic acid and dermatan sulphate, with heparan and chondroitin sulphates as minor components. Although the glycosaminoglycans as a whole constitute less than 1% of the total dry weight of skin, they have a dramatic effect on the hydration of the tissue, being able to bind up to 1000 times their own weight of water. Some proteoglycans synthesised by skin fibroblasts have been characterised through cDNA cloning of core protein sequences. Two small chondroitin/dermatan sulphate proteoglycans have been identified – biglycan (PG-1), and decorin (PG-11) – which contain two and one chondroitin/dermatan sulphate chains respectively, attached to a core protein of approximately 45 kDa (Table 5.2). The core protein sequences have been assigned a role in molecular interactions with other matrix macromolecules such as collagen and fibronectin. Decorin binds to type I collagen and inhibits fibrillogenesis, while transforming growth factor β stimulates collagen synthesis but inhibits decorin production (Kahari *et al.*, 1991). Decorin is found throughout the dermis, although it stains more in the papillary than the reticular dermis, while cultured papillary dermal fibroblasts express more decorin than fibroblasts cultured from reticular dermis. The core protein of a large chondroitin sulphate proteoglycan, versican, has also been characterised, and found to contain several functional domains, including a hyaluronic acid-binding region, a lectin-like sequence, epidermal growth factor-like repeats, and a complement regulatory protein-like domain.

Cell-associated heparan sulphate proteoglycans have been identified in the dermis. Fibroglycan is an integral membrane proteoglycan, while glypican is linked to the cell surface through a glycosyl phosphatidylinositol anchor, and can therefore be released by phospholipase. Glypican follows a distinct metabolic fate, being shed into the extracellular space, whereas the transmembrane proteoglycan, fibroglycan, is predominantly internalised and degraded.

DEGRADATION

In normal adult skin, proteoglycans and hyaluronate metabolism is in a steady state, in which synthesis is balanced by catabolism, and is highly regulated by the resident cells. The turnover rate varies depending upon the type of proteoglycan and its location. In general, cell surface proteoglycans have a much shorter half-life (4–20 hours) than those of the extracellular matrix (days). The mechanisms involved in extracellular matrix proteoglycan degradation are poorly understood, but most likely involve fibroblast proteases such as stromelysin. Degradation of the proteoglycan protein core would release glycosaminoglycan–peptide fragments which may then be internalised, translocated to lysosomes and the protein and glycosaminoglycan constituents completely depolymerised, or they may reach the general circulation. Proteoglycans in the general circulation are cleared by liver endothelial cells which carry receptors with high affinity for proteoglycans and hyaluronate, and are completely degraded in lysosomes.

The control mechanism for extracellular matrix proteoglycan degradation is unknown, but must involve protease inhibitors, the effect of which may be overcome by high local concentrations of a particular protease. Stromelysin, a metalloproteinase, has been shown to degrade cartilage proteoglycan, and its activity may be inhibited by tissue inhibitors of metalloproteinases (TIMPs). Interestingly, fibroblast collagenase, a highly specific metalloproteinase, degrades the protein core of cartilage proteoglycan. Cell surface proteoglycans may be released from the plasma membrane by limited proteolysis and shed into the extracellular matrix, or they may be internalised and degraded in the lysosomes. The lysosomal degradation of glycosaminoglycans is initiated by endohexosaminidase or endoglucuronidase, and the oligosaccharides cleaved sequentially by exoglycosidases and sulphatases. Heparan sulphate may be degraded in the extracellular matrix by heparanases produced by platelets, activated T-lymphocytes, and by metastatic tumour cells, in which a correlation between heparanase production and metastatic potential has been demonstrated. The enzymes involved are likely to be endoglucuronidases, which produce heparan sulphate fragments that are subsequently endocytosed and degraded further intracellularly.

It appears that a large part of hyaluronate is not degraded in the tissue of origin, but rather is transported to the regional lymph nodes, where it is degraded to monosaccharide units. Approximately 10% escapes degradation in the lymph nodes and enters the general circulation. From there it is rapidly taken up into liver sinusoidal endothelial cells by receptor-mediated endocytosis. A small proportion of the circulating hyaluronate is excreted in the urine as small hyaluronate fragments which can penetrate the glomerular basement membrane.

THE MUCOPOLYSACCHARIDOSES

Considerable information has been obtained regarding the metabolism of glycosaminoglycans from studies on the group of human genetic disorders termed the mucopolysaccharidoses (Muenzer, 1986). All are autosomal recessive traits, except for the Hunter syndrome which is sex-linked, and are associated with storage and urinary excretion of excessive amounts of glycosaminoglycans. The type of glycosaminoglycans being stored or excreted is used to classify the mucopolysaccharidoses into subgroups, identified with specific enzyme deficiencies, and these are summarised in Table 5.3. As would be expected with such disorders, defects are not restricted to the skin; they involve connective tissues, skeletal malformations, and are frequently associated with mental retardation. Apart from the marked changes in the appearance of the patients, such as their coarse features, cutaneous changes are not prominent, although the skin is often thickened, and excessive hair growth may occur in several of the disorders.

THE HAIR GROWTH CYCLE

It is now becoming increasingly apparent that epithelial–mesenchymal cell interactions are influenced by changes in extracellular matrix composition, and

Table 5.3. The mucopolysaccharidoses subgroups

Subgroup	Deficient enzyme	GAG affected	Syndrome
MPS I-H	α-Iduronidase	DS, HS	Hurler
MPS I-S	α-Iduronidase	DS, HS	Scheie
MPS II	Iduronate sulphatase	DS, HS	Hunter
MPS III-A	Heparan-N-sulphatase	HS	Sanfilippo A
MPS III-B	α–N-Acetylglucosaminidase	HS	Sanfilippo B
MPS III-C	N-Acetylase	HS	Sanfilippo C
MPS III-D	N-Acetylglucosamine-6-sulphatase	HS	Sanfilippo D
MPS IV-A	Galactose-6-sulphatase	C-6S, KS	Morquio A
MPS IV-B	β-Galactosidase	KS	Morquio B
MPS VI	N-Acetylgalactosamine-4-sulphatase	DS	Maroteaux–Lamy
MPS VII	β-Glucuronidase	DS, C4/6S, HS	Sly

that such changes may be particularly important in regulating hair growth. The first evidence that glycosaminoglycans may be involved in hair growth control was the observation of excessive hair growth in some of the mucopolysaccharidoses disorders. In addition, many patients receiving systemic heparin therapy experience hair loss which is dose dependent and reversible. It has now been shown that there are specific changes in the composition and concentrations of glycosaminoglycans in the skin, associated with different stages of the hair growth cycle. The changes are particularly evident in rodents, where the hair cycle is synchronised and clearly defined. Heparin levels in rat skin show a rapid but short-lived peak in anagen, with baseline levels in catagen and telogen, and the number of dermal mast cells also fluctuates. It would therefore appear that the controlled release of heparin from dermal mast cells may be important in the regulation of anagen follicle development.

The basement membrane proteoglycans also change throughout the rat hair growth cycle. Immunohistochemical studies have revealed that during the hair growth cycle heparan sulphate proteoglycan persists around hair follicles, while a basement membrane-specific chondroitin sulphate decreases through catagen until it is undetectable at the base and dermal papillae of the telogen follicle. As anagen recommences, expression of the chondroitin sulphate proteoglycan is again apparent. Similar studies of the human scalp have revealed that during anagen the thick connective tissue sheath around the follicle, and the dermal papillae, stain strongly for chondroitin-6-sulphate, unsulphated chondroitin, and dermatan sulphate. In mid-catagen, the staining for chondroitin-6-sulphate and chondroitin decreases significantly until it is barely detectable by late catagen. Chondroitin-6-sulphate reappears in early anagen.

WOUND HEALING

Cutaneous wound repair provides a complex, highly regulated series of biological events in which we can study the role of proteoglycans and glycosaminoglycans in cellular migration, proliferation, differentiation, and matrix synthesis and assembly.

The sequence begins with the flooding of the wound with blood products, and the formation of a clot of fibrin and fibronectin, together with the initiation of the early phase of inflammation. Mediators released as a result of this initial event stimulate the migration of further inflammatory cells and fibroblasts into the wound area, followed by cellular proliferation and angiogenesis. The granulation tissue that rapidly forms is gradually modified as the wound matures. Re-epithelialisation begins within 24 hours after injury, and continues during the formation of granulation tissue. The initial formation of a fibrin/fibronectin clot, in which fibrin is cross-linked both to itself and to fibronectin by plasma transglutaminase, provides a suitable substrate for cellular migration into the wound space. There, mediators released as a consequence of blood coagulation, complement pathways, and cell activation induce an influx of inflammatory leucocytes. Increasing numbers of macrophages appear, and together with platelets they release several factors crucial for the production of granulation tissue. The major factors include platelet-derived growth factor, fibroblast growth factors, epidermal growth factor, and transforming growth factors α and β. Certain matrix breakdown products are also chemotactic, including collagen, elastin, fibronectin and hyaluronate fragments. Early granulation tissue contains large amounts of fibronectin and hyaluronate, and immature collagen fibrils. While fibronectin may mediate cellular adhesion and migration, hyaluronate also seems to be associated with cell migration and proliferation. The highly hydrated and expanded structure of hyaluronate will ensure that a matrix of low impedance is formed and will allow penetration by ingrowing parenchymal cells.

As the wound matures, not only does most of the abundant fibronectin disappear, but a fall in the hyaluronate level is associated with the appearance of hyaluronidase. Just how the interplay of fibronectin and hyaluronate influences cellular adhesion and migration is unclear. High concentrations of hyaluronate and chondroitin sulphate proteoglycan may reduce cellular adhesion, in particular to fibronectin. Dermal fibroblast adhesion to fibronectin is mediated via cell surface integrin receptors binding to an arginine, glycine, aspartic acid, serine (RGDS) cell-binding sequence in the fibronectin molecule, and adhesion is probably reinforced by the binding of cell surface heparan sulphate proteoglycan to the heparin-binding domain of fibronectin. Hyaluronate may weaken this proteoglycan–fibronectin interaction, and facilitate migration. Tenascin, an extracellular matrix glycoprotein, is known to partially inhibit the attachment of a number of cells to fibronectin, and may therefore complement the effect of hyaluronate. In normal skin, tenascin is expressed just beneath the dermo-epidermal junction, while in healing wounds it is abundant throughout the dermis. The high concentrations of hyaluronate during the period of rapid cellular proliferation are consistent with the finding that cultures of rapidly growing fibroblasts, and indeed many other cell types, produce significantly more hyaluronate than confluent stationary cultures.

Heparan sulphate proteoglycans may also be important in regulating cellular proliferation, which may be mediated not only by quantitative changes but also by modification of the glycosaminoglycan chain substituents. Such a role is suggested by the observation that cell surface heparan sulphate proteoglycan is shed from the cell surface immediately before cell division, while heparan sulphate synthesised by confluent smooth muscle cells will inhibit the growth of subconfluent cells. Proteoglycans may also be important in regulating angiogenesis. Confluent endothelial cells synthesise heparan sulphate proteoglycan, while migrating cells synthesise predominantly chondroitin and dermatan sulphate. Disrupted mast cells, however, release a heparin which is known to be an endothelial cell chemoattractant. Angiogenesis therefore depends not only upon mitogenic and chemotactic factors, but also on the presence of an appropriate proteoglycan-containing extracellular matrix.

Two weeks after injury, as the wound matures, the synthesis of chondroitin-4-sulphate and dermatan sulphate increases but there is a rapid decrease in hyaluronate. These proteoglycans are probably involved in regulating collagen fibrillogenesis, and indeed chondroitin-4-sulphate has been shown to accelerate polymerisation of type I collagen monomers *in vitro*. The large amount of chondroitin sulphate in granulation tissue, but not in mature scar tissue, and elevated collagen synthesis and chondroitin-4-sulphate in hypertrophic scars supports this concept. The small dermatan sulphate proteoglycan decorin is thought to be involved in regulating collagen fibrillogenesis (Scott, 1991). The association of dermatan sulphate proteoglycans with collagen fibrils has been demonstrated using cupromeronic blue. In the electron microscope, collagen fibrils are easily visualised, while the proteoglycans can be stained with cupromeronic blue, which contains a copper atom and therefore enhances its electron density. The stain is also useful in light microscopy; being intensely blue and positively charged, it binds readily to the polyanionic glycosaminoglycans. Using critical electrolyte concentrations of magnesium chloride, its staining of glycosaminoglycans can be made highly specific. Electron microscopy reveals proteoglycans as dark filaments orthogonally and regularly arranged along the collagen fibrils, one D period apart. Using both chemical analysis and specific enzymes, the proteoglycan was identified as being dermatan sulphate. It seems likely therefore that chondroitin-4-sulphate is involved in initial polymerisation of collagen molecules, while dermatan sulphate may modify the formation of collagen fibres and bundles. The interplay of proteoglycans and hyaluronate therefore appears to be critical in regulating cellular adhesion, migration, proliferation, and in the synthesis and assembly of the matrix molecules.

FIBROTIC DISORDERS

Following initiation of an inflammatory phase, there is a normal fibrotic response in healing wounds which progresses through a granulation tissue and matrix remodelling phase and finally results in healed scar tissue that resembles the normal connective tissue. The interplay of several cytokines and growth factors, and the composition of the extracellular matrix, are undoubtedly involved in regulating these phases, but the precise mechanisms remain unclear. Fibroblasts cultured from early phase traumatic wound tissue, or from sites of pathological fibrosis such as keloids or sclerodermatous skin, show increased synthesis of collagens, glycosaminoglycans and fibronectin in the absence of further stimulation, suggesting that some other factors are required to end this synthetic phase. Keloid formation and wound healing share similar histopathological appearances in early stages, but in keloids, as fibroplasia progresses, nodular vascular proliferations appear associated with increased numbers of fibroblasts, and eventually form thickened nodular masses of collagen and proteoglycan. Keloids have been differentiated from hypertrophic scars, but both conditions are characterised by striking increases in glycosaminoglycan levels compared to normal skin. Collagen fibre formation also appears to be disrupted, and keloids contain collagen bundles and fibres that are haphazard and loosely connected. Total glycosaminoglycan levels, and especially hyaluronate, are elevated, while the proportion of chondroitin-4-sulphate is increased. These changes in glycosaminoglycan levels and composition may contribute to the abnormal collagen fibrillogenesis. Fibroblasts cultured from hypertrophic scar are similar in growth rate and protein synthesis to normal skin fibroblasts or those isolated from normal scar tissue. Hypertrophic scar fibroblasts, however, synthesise substantially more hyaluronate and chondroitin sulphate than control cells, and therefore reflect to some extent the glycosaminoglycan changes observed *in vivo*.

Sclerodermatous disorders are characterised by dermal hardening, but the spectrum of these diseases ranges from localised scleroderma (morphoea), where the emphasis is on dermal thickening, to progressive systemic sclerosis, in which fibrotic changes in the skin, blood vessels and internal organs involve the massive deposition of collagen. Immunohistochemical staining of skin proteoglycans in patients with systemic sclerosis reveals vascular proteoglycans in early lesions which is later replaced by deposition between the collagen fibres, suggesting a vascular initiation of the skin lesion. The pathogenesis of the disease therefore appears to involve factors from plasma or platelets which, upon diffusion into the dermis or other tissues, may stimulate matrix synthesis by fibroblasts. Scleroderma fibroblasts are also more responsive to certain growth factors than normal fibroblasts: they synthesise more glycosaminoglycans in response to a platelet release fraction, transforming growth factor β and mitogen-activated T-lymphocytes (Falanga et al., 1987). Lesional skin contains more glycosaminoglycans, particularly in the early oedematous phase of the disease, and there also appears to be a compositional change, with increased synthesis of dermatan sulphate. Patients with systemic scleroderma also have raised serum hyaluronate and urinary sulphated glycosaminoglycans. Interestingly, a heparan sulphate-like glycosaminoglycan isolated from the urine of systemic scleroderma patients induces a scleroderma-like response in mice when injected intraperitoneally.

Another disorder characterised by excessive synthesis of glycosaminoglycans is pretibial myxoedema. In this relatively rare disorder there is localised thickening of the skin, with excessive production of hyaluronic acid and separation of collagen fibres. The pathogenesis is unknown; however, when normal skin fibroblasts are exposed to serum from patients with pretibial myxoedema, they produce increased amounts of hyaluronate. According to one study, fibroblasts from lower extremities appear to be more sensitive to the serum-derived fibroblast-stimulating factor, and produce more hyaluronate than fibroblasts from other areas, which may explain why localised myxoedema is predominantly found in the pretibial area.

TUMOUR INVASION

There is a striking similarity between some of the processes involved in both wound healing and tumour growth and invasion. Growth of solid tumours requires the active participation of various normal cells such as fibroblasts, vascular endothelial cells, smooth muscle cells, and possibly cells of the immune system – cells similarly involved in wound healing. In addition, wound healing and tumour stroma generation share a number of features, including hyperpermeable blood vessels from which the deposition of a fibrin–fibronectin gel results, providing a provisional matrix which will later be replaced by granulation tissue. While proteoglycans and glycosaminoglycans play important parts in the wound-healing process, with substantial changes in the amounts of hyaluronate and chondroitin/dermatan sulphate proteoglycans, these glycosaminoglycans are also more abundant in and around solid tumours. Indeed it is increasingly clear that a change in tissue architecture occurs around many growing and invading tumours, which may facilitate the invasion of the tissue by tumour cells or aid vascularisation.

The altered glycosaminoglycan composition of the extracellular matrix in healing wounds and tumour stroma may stimulate cell migration, and also facilitate cell growth, as, for example, hyaluronate has been found to modulate cell proliferation. Many tumours have greater amounts of hyaluronate and chondroitin sulphate proteoglycan in their surrounding tissue, and many tumour cell lines synthesise more hyaluronate *in vitro* than their normal counterparts. However, most of the hyaluronate surrounding tumours appears to be synthesised by resident fibroblasts, possibly stimulated by tumour-derived factors. Many of the fibroblast-mediated changes in the extracellular matrix of healing wounds are stimulated by factors derived from inflammatory cells, and while these substances may also be present in tumour stroma, tumour cells undoubtedly release factors which stimulate normal cells to modify the surrounding tissue.

Co-cultures of colon carcinoma cells and smooth muscle cells produce significantly more hyaluronate and chondroitin sulphate proteoglycan than the sum of the individual cultures, while skin fibroblasts cultured from some breast cancer patients release factor(s) into the culture medium that stimulate hyaluronate synthesis by normal skin fibroblasts (Schor *et al.*, 1989). As in several skin disorders associated with excessive dermal glycosaminoglycan synthesis, hyaluronate is significantly increased in the serum of patients with metastatic breast cancer. Indeed dermal fibroblasts cultured from such patients produce a factor that stimulates both the migration of normal adult fibroblasts into collagen gels and their synthesis of hyaluronate. Excised basal cell carcinoma tissue releases factors into culture medium, as do human metastatic melanoma cells, that stimulate hyaluronate synthesis by adult skin fibroblasts greater than tenfold. Incorporation of [^{3}H]glucosamine into sulphated glycosaminoglycans is also enhanced, but to a lesser extent, while $^{35}SO_4$ incorporation remains unchanged, suggesting that the degree of sulphation is reduced. Culture medium conditioned by murine B16 melanoma cells also stimulates fibroblast hyaluronate synthesis, while the B16 tumour cells themselves do not synthesise hyaluronate. In addition, the molecular weight of fibroblast hyaluronate is substantially increased following stimulation by tumour cell-derived factors. Another interesting feature of growing and invading tumours is the expression of tenascin in the surrounding matrix, similar to that found in granulation tissue.

Immunohistochemical staining for chondroitin sulphate proteoglycan and the dermatan sulphate proteoglycan decorin has been examined in healing wounds, normal skin, and in both basal cell and squamous cell carcinomas, in which the antibodies are directed against the chondroitin sulphate chains and the decorin core protein respectively (Yeo *et al.*, 1991). Normal skin stains weakly for chondroitin sulphate and strongly for decorin while, in contrast, wound granulation tissue and tumour stroma stain intensely for chondroitin sulphate and very weakly for decorin. However, decorin staining is restored following digestion with chondroitinase ABC, suggesting that decorin antigenic sites had been masked by glycosaminoglycan chains. Some of the factors mediating the healing response are probably similar to those released by growing and invading tumours. Fibroblasts dispersed within a collagen gel and incubated with serum contract the gel into a tissue-like lattice. In serum-free medium, a number of factors have been shown to stimulate contraction, including transforming growth factor β (TGFβ), medium from endothelial cell cultures and, recently, factors released by basal cell carcinomas and malignant melanomas.

AGEING

Ageing may be regarded as a cellular process that is partly genetically determined and partly influenced by endogenous and exogenous wear and tear. Cutaneous ageing is characterised by a decrease in functional capacity and an increased susceptibility to certain diseases and environmental insults. The most obvious changes include wrinkling, laxity, dryness, general thinning, and a flattening of the dermal/epidermal interface resulting from the retraction of the epidermal papillae and the microprojections of basal cells into the dermis. The three-dimensional arrangement of dermal collagen and elastin fibres shows marked changes in aged skin, becoming more compact, possibly due to changes in the proteoglycans and hyaluronate. Many of the collagen bundles appear to unravel and elastic fibres are fewer and fragmented.

Age-related changes in dermal collagen and elastin have been extensively studied, including those in UV-aged skin, but few changes in glycosamino-glycans have been reported. Hyaluronate, the predominant glycosamino-glycan in early developing dermis, decreases rapidly with age, while the amount of dermatan sulphate increases. Hyaluronate and, not surprisingly, water content, are high throughout the fetal period, but decline rapidly to adult levels by approximately 6 months after birth. There appears to be a slight but gradual decrease in the content of glycosaminoglycans, and in particular hyaluronate, with increasing age, and while glycosaminoglycans may be a minor component of the dry weight, such a decrease may adversely affect the skin's turgor and ability to dissipate compressive forces, as glycosaminog-lycans bind immense volumes of water. Glycosaminoglycan changes in ageing rat skin are summarised in Fig. 5.3. In addition to thinning and reduced hyaluronate and dermatan sulphate content, elderly skin is relatively acellular and avascular. In particular, mast cells in the papillary dermis are substantially fewer compared to young adults. Such a reduction may result in decreased levels of mast cell-derived heparin, which in turn may be involved in angiogenesis. The ageing of dermal fibroblasts *in vitro*, that is, the changes appearing after several passages, involves a decline in the synthesis of hyaluronate and dermatan sulphate, but such decreases may also be associated with the ageing cell's declining proliferation rate.

It is important that studies of chronological ageing are performed on sun-protected skin, as there are marked differences between such aged skin and actinically damaged dermis. Photo-ageing changes in skin include injury to

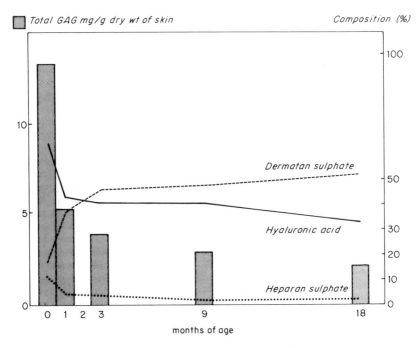

Fig. 5.3. Age-related changes in glycosaminoglycans (GAG) in the skin of the rat

basal keratinocytes, resulting in a scaly horny layer and multiple actinic keratoses, and frequently epidermal atrophy, possibly due to depletion of the germinative layer. Prominent wrinkling is probably caused by changes in collagen and elastin fibres and possibly in glycosaminoglycans. There is an accumulation of elastotic material, and increased staining for glycosamino-glycans, while biochemical analysis has confirmed an increased glycosamino-glycan, but lower collagen content. There is probably progressive injury to dermal fibroblasts in sun-exposed skin, with a resultant change in their extracellular matrix synthesis, although the presence of a lymphocytic infiltrate in chronically sun-exposed skin may contribute to the observed matrix changes through the release of degradative enzymes and inflammatory mediators.

The skin of hairless mice exposed to UV irradiation also shows thickened elastic fibres, a loss of collagen, and increased amounts of glycosaminoglycans (Schwartz, 1988). Topical treatment of photo-aged skin with all-*trans*-retinoic acid has, in many cases, improved the clinical and histological appearance of the damaged skin, the improvements including a thicker epidermis, less wrinkling, enhanced vascularity, and deposition of new collagen. Retinoic acid inhibits collagenase activity and hyaluronate synthesis by skin fibroblasts *in vitro*, but also enhances the production of the collagenase inhibitor TIMP.

PSORIASIS

Surprisingly little is known about the pathogenesis of psoriasis, a disorder originally considered to be a disease of the epidermis, but now known to involve the dermis and sites outside the skin. The disease is characterised by red scaly patches, inflammation and keratinocyte hyperproliferation, turnover being reduced from approximately 4 weeks to as little as 3 days. However, keratinocyte hyperproliferation is also apparent in adjacent uninvolved skin. The signals for epidermal cell hyperproliferation are unknown, but low calcium concentrations stimulate proliferation in cultured keratinocytes, suggesting a possible role for the recently identified calcium-binding protein osteonectin, or perhaps calmodulin, by reducing extracellular free calcium in psoriatic epidermis. Their presence in such lesions has not yet been examined, but supporting this theory is the observation that osteonectin is present in the migrating epidermal tongue in healing wounds, but is absent from normal epidermis.

There is increasing evidence that the dermis plays an important role in the aetiology of psoriasis. Dermal abnormalities include increases in prolyl hydroxylase activity and collagen solubility, altered glycosaminoglycan staining, and capillary dilation and tortuosity. Increased synthesis of glycosaminoglycans, and in particular hyaluronate, seems likely, but there are few reports on the content and composition of glycosaminoglycans from psoriatic skin. Just how glycosaminoglycan changes would influence epidermal turnover is unclear, but increased levels of hyaluronate are observed during morphogenetic cell migrations, during wound healing and in the matrix surrounding many growing and invading tumours. In addition, expression of the glycoprotein tenascin is substantially elevated in the dermis of psoriatic lesions, and during wound healing. Further evidence for an increased content of hyaluronate in the dermis is the considerable rise in hyaluronate in suction blister fluid from involved skin compared to that from control or uninvolved skin.

Much of the current information on glycosaminoglycan changes in psoriasis has come from studies of cultured fibroblasts, which suggest a defect in the dermis. Cultured psoriatic fibroblasts show an increase in proliferation rate, collagen and general protein synthesis, and glycosaminoglycan synthesis. However, such studies are complicated by the fact that glycosaminoglycan synthesis is affected by cellular growth rate and density, although the increased secretion of glycosaminoglycans by psoriatic fibroblasts is most marked at high cell density. A means of overcoming such growth-related influences might be to examine fibroblast glycosaminoglycan synthesis within contracted collagen lattices, in which fibroblast growth is minimal, although psoriatic fibroblasts might grow better in such matrices than normal cells.

The distribution and composition of glycosaminoglycans in body fluids such as urine and serum have provided valuable information regarding the widespread extracutaneous involvement of the disease, and hints as to where the major defect may lie. Urine from patients with generalised plaque psoriasis contains substantially elevated levels of chondroitin sulphate, which is found in only small amounts in the dermis, suggesting that perhaps tissues rich in this glycosaminoglycan such as bone and cartilage may be the source rather than skin (Priestley, 1988). Indeed successful topical treatment or Psoralen-UVA does not affect the excessive levels of glycosaminoglycan in the urine. As inflammatory events precede epidermal proliferation, infiltration of psoriatic lesions with leucocytes including neutrophils, lymphocytes and monocytes/ macrophages will undoubtedly cause the release of growth factors, which may affect glycosaminoglycan synthesis or turnover directly.

PROTEOGLYCANS AND GROWTH FACTOR ACTIVITIES

The suggestion a number of years ago that proteoglycans might modulate the activities of certain growth factors was probably based on the ability of heparan sulphate proteoglycan and heparin to bind fibroblast growth factors (FGFs). In fact, heparin affinity columns are now frequently used to purify several different growth factors. Growth factors that bind to heparin and heparan sulphate proteoglycans include, in addition to the FGFs, interleukin 3, granulocyte–macrophage colony stimulating factor, pleiotrophin and platelet factor 4. Other proteoglycans are possibly involved in modulating growth factor activity, such as platelet α-granule chondroitin sulphate proteoglycan, which binds platelet factor 4, and a number of small dermatan sulphate proteoglycans which bind to TGFβ.

Heparin augments the mitogenic activity of acidic FGF twentyfold, apparently by extending the factor's half-life from 15 minutes to 26 hours, but there is no comparable synergistic effect of heparin on basic FGF (bFGF). However, involvement of cell surface proteoglycans in bFGF activity is confirmed by the observation that Chinese hamster ovary cells that express the FGF receptor, but cannot synthesise heparan sulphate proteoglycan, do not bind bFGF. Addition of heparin to the culture medium facilitates bFGF binding to its high-affinity receptor (Yayon et al., 1991). It therefore appears that cell surface heparan sulphate proteoglycan provides a cell surface-bound reservoir of the bFGF, while binding of the bFGF to the proteoglycan may cause a conformational change in the growth factor, enabling it to bind to the receptor.

Another theory is that the binding of bFGF to heparan sulphate proteoglycan may affect its oligomerisation in such a way as to cause dimerisation of the receptors, which is thought to be necessary for signal transduction by other receptor tyrosine kinases. While syndecan is a possible candidate for a cell surface FGF-binding proteoglycan, other extracellular matrix proteoglycans undoubtedly bind FGFs, forming an extracellular reservoir of the growth factors. Such immobilised and inactivated FGF may play an important part in processes such as wound healing and tumour invasion. The growth factors bound to extracellular matrix may be released in an active form when extracellular matrix heparan sulphate is degraded, such as by the heparanase expressed by normal cells, including platelets and neutrophils, and by tumour cells, thereby stimulating angiogenesis and tumour cell growth. The binding of the FGFs to the extracellular matrix, and their release by specific enzymes, may therefore provide highly localised control of their activities.

The activity of TGFβ also appears to be modulated by proteoglycans, but unlike the growth factor–proteoglycan interactions previously discussed, TGFβ interacts with the protein core and not the glycosaminoglycan side chains. A cell surface proteoglycan, betaglycan, which contains both heparan and dermatan sulphate chains, has been identified as a low-affinity receptor for TGFβ. Binding of TGFβ to betaglycan may be necessary for its subsequent delivery to the signal-transducing receptor. As with the FGFs, TGFβ also binds to extracellular matrix proteoglycans such as decorin – a small dermatan sulphate proteoglycan. The binding to its core protein appears to neutralise the activity of TGFβ, possibly by competing with the cell surface receptors.

CONCLUDING REMARKS

Proteoglycans are a very heterogeneous group of molecules involved in highly diverse biological processes in which both the protein cores and the glycosaminoglycan chains participate. Such functions will only be fully understood when we know the exact structure of both the core proteins and the glycosaminoglycan chains, and see how their synthesis is regulated. A number of core proteins have been characterised utilising defined cDNAs, and the development of further probes and antibodies will enable the characterisation of many more. Improved methods of glycosaminoglycan sequence analysis will be developed, and should permit correlations to be made between the fine structure of the polysaccharide chains and their biological activity in the near future.

REFERENCES

Brown TA, Bouchard T, St John T, Wayner E and Carter WG (1991) Human keratinocytes express a new CD44 core protein (CD44E) as a heparan sulphate intrinsic membrane proteoglycan with addition exons. *Journal of Cell Biology* **113**, 207–221.
Falanga V, Tiegs SL, Alstadt MS, Roberts AB and Sporn MB (1987) Transforming growth factor-beta: selective increase in glycosaminoglycan synthesis by cultures of fibroblasts from patients with progressive systemic sclerosis. *Journal of Investigative Dermatology* **89**, 100–104.
Kahari V-M, Larjava H and Uitto J (1991) Differential regulation of extracellular matrix proteoglycan (PG) gene expression. *Journal of Biological Chemistry* **266**, 10608–10615.

Muenzer J (1986) Mucopolysaccharidoses. *Advances in Pediatrics* **223**, 209–220.

Priestley GC (1988) Urinary excretion of glycosaminoglycans in psoriasis. *Archives of Dermatological Research* **280**, 77–82.

Schor SL, Schor AM, Grey A-M, Chen J, Rushton G, Grant ME and Ellis I (1989) Mechanism of action of the migration-stimulating factor produced by foetal and cancer patient fibroblasts: effect on hyaluronic acid synthesis. *In Vitro Cellular and Developmental Biology* **25**, 737–746.

Schwartz E (1988) Connective tissue alterations in the skin of ultraviolet irradiated hairless mice. *Journal of Investigative Dermatology* **91**, 158–161.

Scott JE (1991) Proteoglycans: collagen interactions in connective tissues. Ultrastructural, biochemical, functional and evolutionary aspects. *International Journal of Biological Macromolecules* **13**, 157–161.

Tammi R, Ripellino JA, Margolis RU, Maibach HI and Tammi M (1989) Hyaluronate accumulation in human epidermis treated with retinoic acid in skin organ culture. *Journal of Investigative Dermatology* **92**, 326–332.

Yayon A, Klagsbrun M, Esko JD, Leder P and Ornitz DM (1991) Cell surface, heparin-like molecules are required for binding of basic fibroblast growth factor to its high affinity receptor. *Cell* **64**, 841–848.

Yeo T-K, Brown L and Dvorak HF (1991) Alterations in proteoglycan synthesis common to healing wounds and tumours. *American Journal of Pathology* **138**, 1437–1450.

FURTHER READING

Clark RAF (1991) Cutaneous wound repair. In: Goldsmith LA (ed.) *Physiology, Biochemistry and Molecular Biology of the Skin*, 2nd edn, pp. 576–601. Oxford: Oxford University Press.

Couchman JR and Hook M (1988) Proteoglycans and wound repair. In: Clark RAF and Henson PM (eds) *Molecular and Cellular Biology of Wound Repair*, pp. 437–470. London: Plenum Press.

Goetinck PF and Winterbottom N (1991) Proteoglycans: modular macromolecules of the extracellular matrix. In: Goldsmith LA (ed.) *Physiology Biochemistry, and Molecular Biology of the Skin*, 2nd edn, pp. 558–575. Oxford: Oxford University Press.

Hay ED (ed.) (1991) *Cell Biology of Extracellular Matrix*, 2nd edn. New York: Plenum.

Kjellen L and Lindahl U (1991) Proteoglycans: structures and interactions. *Annual Review of Biochemistry* **60**, 443–475.

Ruoslahti E (1988) Structure and biology of proteoglycans. *Annual Review of Cell Biology* **4**, 229–255.

Ruoslahti E and Yamaguchi Y (1991) Proteoglycans as modulators of growth factor activities. *Cell* **64**, 867–869.

6 Dermal Proteins and their Degradative Enzymes

J.B. WEISS

The macromolecular composition of skin is extremely complex. This chapter covers only the structural proteins of the dermis, such as the collagens and elastins, and the enzymes which are able to degrade them. Although these proteins constitute a large part of the skin, they do not include fibronectin and proteoglycans, for example, or all the basement membrane proteins, which are covered in other chapters.

During the past 5 years there has been an enormous increase in our knowledge of some of the minor collagens and of elastin and its associated fibrillar protein. This chapter attempts to bring the reader up to date with these recent discoveries.

COLLAGEN

At the time of writing this chapter there are 14 officially numbered types of collagen, with perhaps more waiting in the wings, yet to be given an official number. Fortunately for the reader only eight of these collagens are currently known to be present in skin and some may think that is enough. Although these collagens differ in the manner of their polymeric assembly, they have many similarities in their primary molecular structure. All collagen molecules consist of three polypeptide chains known as α chains, each of which coil in a left-handed minor helix. The three chains then coil together into a triple or super helix. In some types of collagen the chains of the triple helix have identical amino acid sequences, in others they differ. Some collagens contain molecules which are predominantly triple helical, having only small amino acid and carboxy terminal non-helical regions. In others the triple helical conformation is interrupted along the molecule by non-helical intermolecular regions and/or large non-helical terminal globular domains. Helical regions are given the nomenclature [COL] and non-helical regions the nomenclature [NC].

Helical regions of protein [COL] consist of repeating triplets of amino acids of which every third residue is glycine. The Gly–X–Y triplet has a high content

Molecular Aspects of Dermatology. Edited by G.C. Priestley.
© 1993 by John Wiley & Sons Ltd

Table 6.1. Molecular formulae and nature of aggregation of the skin collagens

Type	Nature of aggregates	Molecular formula
I[a]	Fibrils	$[\alpha 1(I)]_2 \alpha 2(I)$
III	Fibrils	$[\alpha 1(III)]_3$
V	Fibrils	$[\alpha 1(V)]_2 \alpha 2(V)$
IV	Networks (basement membranes)	$[\alpha 1(IV)]_2 \alpha 2(IV)$
VI	Macrofibrils	$\alpha 1(VI) \alpha 2(VI) \alpha 3(VI)$
VII	Anchoring fibrils	$[\alpha 1(VII)]_3$
XII[b]	FACIT	$[\alpha 1(XII)]_3$
XIV[b]	FACIT	$[\alpha 1(XIV)]_3$

[a] A very minor form of type I collagen, type I trimer $[\alpha 1(I)]_3$, has been described in fetal skin.
[b] FACIT = fibril associated collagens with interrupted triple helices.

of the imino acids proline and hydroxyproline. The proline residues when present are usually in the X-position and hydroxyproline in the Y position. Hydroxyproline arises as a product of post-translational modification of the *in situ* proline residue. This is one of many post-translational modifications which occur in collagen, others being hydroxylation of some lysine residues, with subsequent attachment of a galactose residue to some of these. A glucose residue may also be attached to a galactose residue but like other modifications this is not inevitable. The enzymes involved in these processes are prolyl and lysyl hydroxylases, and galactosyl and glucosyl transferases. The modifications take place within the cell but further extracellular modifications may occur after secretion of the procollagen molecule. These changes may involve processing of the terminal propeptide and the oxidative deamination of the amino groups in specific lysyl or hydroxylysyl residues by the enzyme lysyl oxidase, a metalloenzyme containing copper, which must be in the Cu(II) state for activity. The lysyl or hydroxylysyl aldehydes derived from this treatment take part in the formation of cross-links which give strength to the collagen fibrils. As mentioned earlier, the constituent chains of the various types of collagen may be genetically distinct or identical within each molecule. Table 6.1 shows the molecular configuration and nature of the α chains of the collagens of skin.

TYPES I, III AND V COLLAGENS

Of the eight types of collagen in skin only three – types I, III and V – are fibrillar collagens exhibiting the typical banded pattern seen in electron microscopy. These collagens are further processed extracellularly by removal of their non-triple helical [NC] terminal procollagen extensions by amino and carboxy terminal propeptidases specific for each collagen type. Subsequently the molecules assemble into approximately a quarter-stagger register (actually 67 nm), with gaps and overlap regions as shown diagrammatically in Fig. 6.1. Although collagen types I and III can both form fibrils on their own *in vitro*, it appears that *in vivo* the two molecules become part of the same fibril, and it has

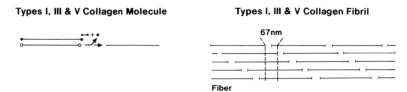

Fig. 6.1. Diagrammatic representation of type I collagen molecule showing the nature of the assembly into fibrils. Reprinted from Uitto and Perejda (1987) p. 116 by courtesy of Marcel Dekker Inc.

recently been shown that skin fibrils are heterotypic, consisting of both type I and type III collagens. Covalent cross-links have also been described between type I and types III and V collagen molecules. However, it may be of interest that when extracting collagen from skin, an initial neutral salt extraction removes types I, III and V collagen, although in very small amounts, but subsequent acetic acid extraction produces only type I collagen, suggesting an acid-soluble cross-link for type I collagen but not for type III collagen, or that some type I fibrils are not associated with type III collagen fibrils.

The fibrillar collagen in skin consists mainly of types I and III collagen and the ratio of I to III appears to change from fetal to adult skin. In fetal skin it is approximately 1.0 whereas adult skin contains considerably more type I than type III. In both adult and fetal skin type V collagen is a minor component, representing less than 5% of the total collagen. The way in which these three collagen types co-polymerise is not clear. It has been suggested that addition of types III and V collagen to type I collagen limits the fibril diameter quite considerably. This, however, has only been shown in reconstituted fibrils *in vitro*. On the other hand, type V collagen is not easily visualised by immunohistochemistry, unless the collagen fibrils have been swollen artificially, suggesting that this collagen is buried to some extent within the fibril.

Impaired cleavage of the amino terminal propeptide from type I procollagen has been demonstrated in the Ehlers–Danlos syndrome (EDS) type VII. Two abnormalities have been observed: one in which the amino acid sequence at the cleavage site is aberrant and another in which an abnormal procollagen protease has been implicated (Kivirikko and Kuivaniemi, 1987). These patients have soft, non-fragile skin which is mildly hyperextensible. In type IV EDS there is a reduced or absent synthesis or secretion of type III collagen. The dermis in these patients is thinner than normal; the collagen figrils are small or of variable diameter and there are excessive numbers of elastic fibres (Fig. 6.2). The reason for the latter effect is unknown.

In many of the EDS types, collagen fibrils of abnormal diameter are observed. It has been suggested, on the basis of immunohistochemistry, that the fine filaments observed in the deep subcutaneous tissue of patients with scleroderma are type III collagen (Fleischmajer *et al.*, 1991). However, this now seems unlikely and it is possible that the antibody used was contaminated with type VI collagen. In many of the other EDS subtypes the fibrils are of variable

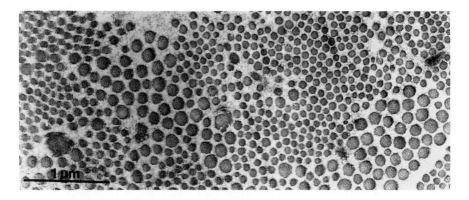

Fig. 6.2. Electron micrograph of dermis from a patient with EDS IV showing variable diameter fibrils. Reprinted from Uitto and Perejda (1987) p. 116 by courtesy of Marcel Dekker Inc.

or large diameter but the reasons for this are only clear in the case of EDS type VI, where there is a deficiency or absence of the enzyme lysyl hydroxylase. This leads to underhydroxylation of lysine residues in types I and III collagens, and since some hydroxylysine residues are also glycosylated, these collagens will be underglycosylated too. Because hydroxylysine residues are involved in cross-linking of collagen, some lack of cross-links may be responsible for the variable diameter. Deficiencies in collagen cross-linking also occur in EDS IX and in Menkes' syndrome, where altered copper metabolism results in loss of activity of lysyl oxidase.

TYPE IV COLLAGEN

Type IV collagen is a major component of basement membranes. Like type I collagen it is a heterotrimer made up of two $\alpha 1$ chains and one $\alpha 2$ chain, $[\alpha 1(IV)]2\ \alpha 2(IV)$. Although in some tissues, such as kidney, type IV collagen has a multiplicity of chains, namely α-III, α-IV and α-V, these do not appear to be present in skin. The propeptides of type IV collagen are not processed and it is assembled as the procollagen form. The molecules are longer than the fibrillar collagens, with at least five interruptions in the triple helix. At the amino terminal end there is a domain known as the 7S domain which comprises both collagenous and non-collagenous regions. Four triple helical domains in this region from four different molecules assemble laterally head to tail and form a spider-like structure, the overlap region being stabilised by disulphide- and lysine-derived cross-links (Fig. 6.3). A sheet-like aggregate is formed by the linking of the carboxy terminal [NC1] domains of the 'spider's legs' to form dimers. Other associations between molecules via their central helical regions have also been described, thus enabling a mesh-like configuration of the polymer to be achieved (Burgeson and Morris, 1987). This collagenous

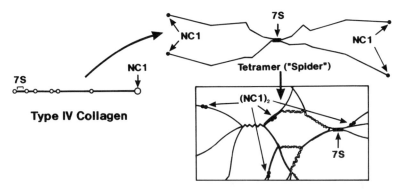

Fig. 6.3. Diagrammatic representation of the type IV collagen molecule and its assembly showing the 7S region and carboxy terminal cross-links. The area within the box shows the assembly of carboxy terminal and 7S cross-linking which occurs *in vivo*. Reproduced from Van der Rest and Garrone (1991) by permission of the Federation of American Societies for Experimental Biology

network of mesh forms the basis for the basement membrane, which is discussed in Chapter 4.

TYPE VI COLLAGEN

Type VI collagen is unique in forming bead-like filaments instead of fibrils. It is a short-chain molecule which associates first into dimers and then the dimers themselves dimerise into a tetrameric form. The non-collagenous regions at each end of the helical chains are not processed, but are incorporated into the filaments, and this explains the bead-like conformation seen in the electron microscope. Recently Kielty *et al.* (1991) have extracted intact collagen type VI microfibrils from calf skin using a novel extraction technique based on the resistance of type VI collagen to bacterial collagenase. Rotary shadowing of the intact extracted microfibrils showed them to be highly flexible and frequently associated with thin-stranded macromolecules that were thought to be hyaluronan (Fig. 6.4). These extracted microfibrils, which were identified by western blotting, had a propensity for lateral association into filamentous structures. As the network of filaments is closely associated with the classical collagen fibrils seen in skin, these authors suggested that they play a role as an interface between the collagen fibril and the fibroblasts, although there is no real evidence for this. It is also suggested that type VI microfibrils are ideally suited to a central role in cell matrix communications, having a capacity to enmesh and possibly interact directly with a range of matrix components, including collagen fibrils, hyaluronan and proteoglycans as well as with the cells themselves. The beaded filaments have repeats of approximately 110 nm.

Type VI collagen has been found in considerably increased amounts in cultured fibroblasts from patients with cutis laxa, and perhaps an excess of type

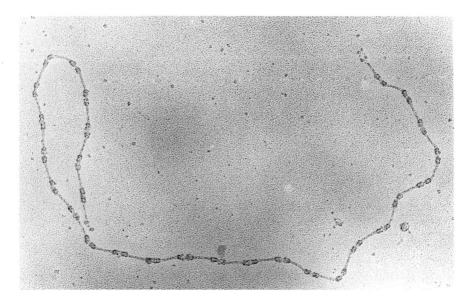

Fig. 6.4. Electron micrograph of rotary shadowed type VI collagen extracted from fetal skin. Courtesy of Dr C. Kielty, Department of Biochemistry, Manchester University

VI collagen may contribute towards the loss of skin elasticity characteristic of this condition. Genes coding for the chains have been mapped to the extremity of the long arm of chromosome 21 and this region is the minimal region of triplication required for the expression of the phenotype of Down's syndrome in partial trisomy 21. It has been suggested that the marked connective tissue abnormalities, such as the hypermobile joints seen in Down's syndrome, are related in some part to type VI collagen (Van der Rest and Garrone, 1991).

TYPE VII COLLAGEN

Type VII collagen is perhaps one of the more interesting types of collagens to the dermatologist, since it is the collagen of the anchoring fibril which is of vital importance in the adherence of the basement membrane of the epithelium to the dermis. Absence or abnormalities of type VII collagen and loss of the anchoring fibrils are thought to be responsible for the blisters caused by separation of epithelial basement membrane from dermis under mild mechanical stress, such as occurs in recessive dystrophic epidermolysis bullosa.

Type VII collagen is a homotrimer. The molecule is made up of a long discontinuous triple helical region that can be spliced with pepsin digestion into two fragments of 94 and 76 kDa per chain respectively. The amino terminal end contains a large non-triple helical non-collagenous domain [NC1] (Fig. 6.5). In some reports the NC1 domain has been ascribed to the carboxy

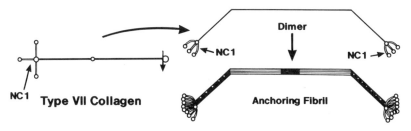

Fig. 6.5. Diagrammatic representation of the type VII collagen molecule showing the assembly into anchoring fibrils. Reproduced from Van der Rest and Garrone (1991) by permission of the Federation of American Societies for Experimental Biology

terminal region of the molecule but this has recently been shown to be incorrect: it is in fact at the amino terminal end (Parente *et al.*, 1991). The molecules assemble into anti-parallel dimers that overlap by 60 nm and are stabilised by at least two intermolecular disulphide bonds. The carboxy terminal [NC2] domain is cleaved, allowing the dimers to aggregate laterally in a non-staggered manner, probably by triple helix interactions. The amino terminal [NC1] domains appear as trident-like shapes, suggesting that a single chain contributes to the structure of each arm and that the three arms are extended (Fig. 6.5). These arms are thought to be capable of individual interactions with basement membrane components, perhaps enabling trivalent interaction of type VII collagen with various macromolecules (Bachinger *et al.*, 1990).

Unlike the other collagens of the dermis and epidermis, type VII collagen is synthesised by keratinocytes and not by fibroblasts. Some collagens such as type IV are synthesised by both fibroblasts and keratinocytes. The overlap of the dimers appears to be an interaction between the [NC2] domain with the triple helix and is stabilised by at least two intermolecular disulphide bonds. It is at this stage that the [NC2] domains are removed and the dimers assemble into anchoring fibrils by unstaggered lateral associations (Fig. 6.5). Anchoring fibrils appear to originate in the lamina densa and to extend into the dermal stroma where they end in anchoring plaques which are basement membrane-like electron-dense regions containing type IV collagen and other basement membrane proteins. The flexibility of the anchoring fibril is through its collagenous regions and not through the claw-like non-collagenous amino terminals.

TYPES XII AND XIV COLLAGENS

Skin also contains two other types of collagen which have been given the nomenclature FACIT collagens (fibril-associated collagens with interrupted triple helices). The recently described types XII and XIV collagen have been demonstrated in bovine skin but their function is unclear at the moment. Type XII collagen is a homotrimer with only two collagenous domains, [COL1] and

[COL2], and a very large non-helical amino terminal section. Rotary shadowing reveals a cross-shaped molecule (Fig. 6.6). There is considerable sequence homology between types XII and XIV collagen and indeed there is some homology in both collagenous and non-collagenous portions with another FACIT collagen found in cartilage (type IX collagen). The [COL1] region of chick type XII has 50% homology with chick α1(IX) [COL1] and although the [COL2] domains are dissimilar, the [NC3] domain of α1(XII) shares 46% nucleotide identity with the [NC4] domain of α1(IX) (Keene *et al.*, 1991). It appears that FACIT collagens, which are considerably shorter and smaller than the fibrillar collagens, lie on the outside of the fibril and may be involved in giving the fibril a function other than that of a scaffolding with tensile strength. Type XII collagen has been located at the surface of type I collagen in calf skin and it has been suggested that the non-helical domains extend outwards from the fibril, while triple helical domains may bind directly to the fibril surface.

The role of these minor collagens is unknown but what is clear is that in the same way that a minor collagen, such as type V, is associated with type I collagen, another minor collagen, type XI, is associated with cartilage type II collagen. Similarly, the FACIT collagen type IX is associated with cartilage collagens and the FACIT collagens XII and XIV with skin and other tissues such as tendon, which contain predominantly type I collagen. These latter collagens are recent additions to the general collagen family and so far no associations have been recorded between them and any disease.

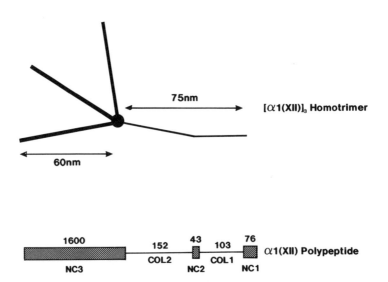

Fig. 6.6. Diagrammatic representation of type XII collagen showing the cross-like structure. Reproduced from Shaw and Olsen (1991) by permission of Elsevier Science Publishers BV

BULLOUS PEMPHIGOID ANTIGEN 2

Very recently the bullous pemphigoid antigen (BP Ag2) has been shown to be a collagen-type protein with non-collagenous sequences (Li et al., 1991). The amino acid sequence, deduced from the cDNA of BP Ag2, has been shown to have a high degree of identity with a recently described cDNA from chicken cornea which had been supposed to encode a cornea-specific collagen. This novel collagen has been mapped by chromosomal in situ hybridisation to the long arm of human chromosome 10. The deduced amino acid sequence for this protein identified two collagenous domains, and the organisation of the exons and supply sites at the intron–exon junction are different from other fibrillar and non-fibrillar collagen genes described to date. There seems to be no association between BP Ag2 and BP Ag1.

ELASTIN

It has long been known from electron micrographic evidence that the elastic fibre consisted of two morphological components: microfibrils and an amorphous component thought to be elastin itself (Ross, 1973). But it is now well established that microfibrils are widely distributed through various connective tissues and are not necessarily associated solely with elastin. However, studies of the microfibrils have revealed two major subgroups and one of these is undoubtedly type VI collagen (see p. 115). The other is a novel protein called fibrillin, which is associated with the amorphous elastin but is also present in the connective tissue network generally (Maddox et al., 1989). In the human dermis the microfibrils are associated with three types of fibres described in older histology literature as oxytalan, elaunin and elastin. The oxytalan fibres present in the capillary layer are anchored to the basal laminar of the epidermo-dermal junction. Oxytalan fibres consist mostly of microfibrils but are thought to contain some elastin, whereas elaunin fibres, which are present beneath the oxytalan fibres, contain both microfibrils and amorphous elastin. However, with the recent elucidation of the nature of the microfibrils as fibrillin and type VI collagen, this concept, based only on staining character-istics, is probably no longer valid.

ELASTIN

The elastic fibres are usually orientated parallel to the epidermis and are mainly of amorphous elastin with small amounts of microfibrils. Elastin itself is a protein which possesses unique elasticity and tensile strength. The strength of the elastin fibres derives from the unusual cross-links desmosine and isodesmosine. These cross-links appear to form spontaneously following enzymatic oxidative deamination of lysine residues (Davies and Anwar, 1970).

The difficulties of discerning the nature of elastin have been partially solved with the discovery of the soluble precursor tropoelastin, which has a molecular mass of approximately 70 kDa and can be extracted from elastin-synthesising tissue such as fetal aorta. This monomeric form of elastin is quite remarkable for its solubility in alcohols and undergoes spontaneous precipitation if it is warmed above 15–20 °C in aqueous solutions. Cross-linking of tropoelastin occurs very rapidly and it is thus rendered an insoluble polymer.

Like collagen, elastin contains approximately 30% glycine in its amino acid composition. It has a somewhat higher proportion of alanine and a remarkably higher proportion of valine. The elastin cross-links are formed in a similar manner to those in collagen by the copper-dependent enzyme lysyl oxidase. Structural analysis of tropoelastin reveals frequent repeat sequences of the pentapeptide PGVGV and the hexapeptide PGVGVA (for key to amino acid notation, see Appendix). These sequences are found in large polypeptides which are generally hydrophobic. Other elastin-derived peptides are rich in lysine and alanine and frequently have polyalanine sequences ending with lysyl residues (AAKAAK): these are thought to represent the domains with the potential for cross-link formation. Skin fibroblasts in culture can be shown to synthesise elastin, but synthesis is highly dependent on cell density and serum concentration.

In human skin one of the characteristics of elastin is its progressive destruction, fragmentation and even disappearance during the course of senescence. It is doubtful whether elastin is newly synthesised in adult organisms except possibly in dermal wound healing. However, increased elastin accumulation in breast tumours and liver fibrosis has been reported.

Several genetic diseases involving elastin are known. Elastoderma is associated with an increased content of the cross-link desmosine in the skin, so that the accumulation of pleomorphic elastic fibres in the lower dermis may be through a failure of elastin degradation. The microfibrils seem to be unaffected. The Buschke–Ollendorff syndrome also involves an increased desmosine content in the skin, but electron microscopy shows an increase of large branching elastic fibres in the dermis and an almost complete loss of the microfibrillar components. The elastic fibres are frequently found near to fibroblastic cells in which the cisternae of the endoplasmic reticulum are dilated. This may indicate an increased production of elastin by such cells. On the other hand, the sparsity of microfibrils may contribute to the faulty assembly of the elastin fibres. The mechanism for the over-production of elastin is not clear but may reflect lack of a feedback control mechanism.

Several cases of cutis laxa have been reported in which the elastic fibres in the dermis were sparse and somewhat fragmented. The reasons for this defect are not known but it may reflect an abnormality of the cross-linking. There is one report of a patient with cutis laxa and an autosomal recessive pulmonary emphysema who had a remarkably elevated activity of serum elastase-like metalloproteinase.

FIBRILLIN

Fibrillin is a large non-collagenous glycoprotein of 350 kDa with intrachain disulphide bonds which assemble into periodic microfibrillar structures (Dahlback *et al.*, 1990). Its synthesis by skin fibroblasts in culture has permitted the production of antibodies and the study of the location of fibrillin in whole tissues. Fibrillin has been shown to be associated with fibrous tissue common to most connective tissues and to be a major component of elastin-associated microfibrils. In a recent very elegant study (Kielty *et al.*, 1991), microfibrils extracted intact from fetal skin were shown to consist of both type VI collagen and fibrillin (see p. 119). In their novel extraction procedure these investigators observed that the fibrillin was easier to extract than the type VI collagen, which required the removal of the majority of collagen fibres before the type VI collagen was released. In Fig. 6.7 the flexibility and branching features of fibrillin can be seen.

A glycoprotein apparently identical to fibrillin was described by Australian

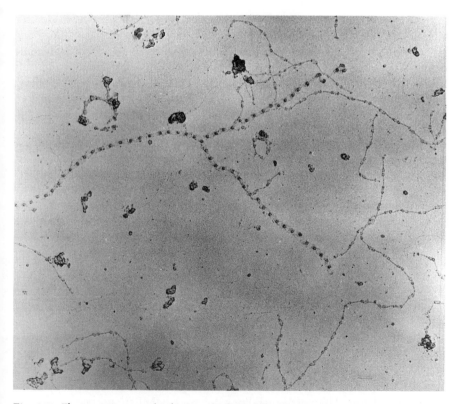

Fig. 6.7. Electron micrograph of rotary shadowed fibrillin microfibrils extracted from fetal skin. Note the extreme flexibility and branching. Courtesy of Dr C. Kielty, Department of Biochemistry, Manchester University

workers (Gibson *et al.*, 1989) and given the name MP 340. Abundant fibrillin microfibrils have been isolated from fetal calf tissues such as skin and aorta and these macromolecules may play a role in the development of such tissues. Immunohistochemical studies on human skin have indicated that fibrillin may form a network that anchors the dermal elastic fibres in the extracellular matrix and to the lamina densa. However, the demonstration by Kielty *et al.* that fibrillin is already abundant in second trimester pre-elastic tissues in the form of a relatively inflexible long branching array suggests the alternative possibility that fibrillin microfibrils exist *in vivo* as coarse networks able to direct and support the subsequent laying down of elastin.

Microfibrils free from amorphous elastin are increased significantly in the subcutaneous skin and lower dermis of patients with both localised and systemic sclerosis. It has been suggested that genes for collagen and microfibrils may be activated simultaneously during fibrosis and perhaps in other biological processes such as development or wound healing (Fleisch-majer *et al.*, 1991). However, it now seems likely that these microfibrils consisted of type VI collagen.

Evidence that fibrillin may be the Marfan gene is of very considerable interest. The immunofluorescence pattern of fibrillin in both tissue (skin) and cell (fibroblast) culture samples from individuals with Marfan's syndrome points to abnormalities of the microfibrillar structure or assembly in this connective tissue disorder. One of the genes for fibrillin has now been localised to chromosome 15 in a position close to that of gene markers linked to Marfan's syndrome, and it is now generally accepted that the abnormality in this syndrome is related to fibrillin and not to collagen as had previously been thought (Lee *et al.*, 1991). Another fibrillin gene located on chromosome 5 has been linked to congenital contractual arachnodactyly.

DEGRADATIVE ENZYMES

COLLAGENASES

Like the collagen components of the dermal matrix, the number and types of the degradative enzymes (collagenases) are also increasing. As some of these enzymes degrade not only collagens but also fibronectin, gelatin and proteoglycans, the term matrix metalloproteinases has been conferred on them. As the term metalloproteinase implies, these enzymes contain an integral metal ion, in this case zinc. They also require calcium as a co-factor and can therefore be inactivated with chelating agents such as ethylenediaminetetraacetic acid (EDTA) and reactivated if calcium is added back to the mixture; although 100% activity will not be restored, as enzyme becomes denatured very easily in the absence of calcium. The matrix metalloproteinases (MMPs) have been numbered from 1 to 10, although for some reason unclear to me types 4, 5 and 6 are missing. Table 6.2 shows the types of metalloproteinases known and their cellular source.

Table 6.2. Matrix metalloproteinases of skin: cellular source and substrate specificity

Name	Cell source	Substrate
MMP-1 (collagenase)	Fibroblasts, endothelial cells	I, II, III collagens
MMP-2 (gelatinase-A)	Fibroblasts	IV, V, VII collagens, fibronectin, gelatin
MMP-3 (stromelysin-1)	Fibroblasts	Proteoglycans, laminin, fibronectin, non-helical regions of IV collagen and procollagens, I, II, III
MMP-8	Polymorphoneutrophils	As MMP-1
MMP-9	Macrophages	As MMP-2
MMP-10	Macrophages	As MMP-3

It is becoming clearer that the MMP family share some distinctive features in their sequence. As Fig. 6.8 illustrates, the signal peptide or pro-domain appears to be identical in these enzymes, which is not surprising as this sequence is required to allow secretion of the finished protein from the cell. The pro-domain which is cleaved when the enzyme is activated contains a highly conserved sequence PRCGVPDV (the key to the one-letter sequence is given in the Appendix to this chapter). Many workers have suggested, but so far not proved, that the cysteine residue in this sequence plays an important role in maintaining the enzyme in the latent form. These enzymes contain several distinct domains which are conserved among the various family members. In the catalytic domain there is a conserved region with three histidine residues which is thought to be the zinc-binding region, since the bacterial metallo-proteinase thermolysin also has conserved histidine residues and contains zinc. Mutations in this region indicate that these residues are required for proteolytic activity. Another domain has sequence similarity with the

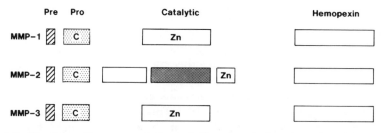

Fig. 6.8. Diagrammatic representation of the shared domains of matrix metallo-proteinases (MMP) 1, 2 and 3. C represents the highly conserved sequence PRCGVPDV (see Appendix) which is believed to play a role in maintaining the enzyme in the latent form. Zn domain is the catalytic domain and contains a conserved region with three histidine residues that is believed to be the zinc binding region (Matrisian, 1990)

Table 6.3. Natural activators of matrix metalloproteinases

Pro-enzyme	Activators
MMP-1	Plasmin, trypsin, MMP-3, ESAF
MMP-2	ESAF
MMP-3	Plasmin, trypsin, ESAF

haem-binding protein haemopexin. Matrix metalloproteinases MMP-2 and -9, which have specificity towards type IV collagen and are sometimes known as basement membrane degrading enzymes or previously as gelatinases, have another domain upstream from the zinc-binding area, and these domains have sequence similarity to the collagen-binding domains of fibronectin. MMP-9 also contains an area identical to type V collagen. The fibronectin domain is believed to be involved in substrate binding of the enzyme.

All the MMPs are secreted from the cell as zymogens and have to be activated in some manner. With the exception of MMP-2, activation is possible through proteolytic digestion. Thus plasmin has been proposed as an activator of these proenzymes, an idea favoured by the fact that in stimulated endothelial cells and fibroblasts MMP-1 and plasmin or plasminogen activator are synthesised and secreted simultaneously in response to cytokine stimulation. However, the activation of pro-MMP-2 is not achievable by any proteinase (Okada *et al.*, 1990). A low-molecular-weight non-protein factor, endothelial cell-stimulating angiogenic factor (ESAF), is able to activate all the pro-matrix metalloproteinases, including MMP-2, and this activity may contribute towards its action as an angiogenic factor (Weiss *et al.*, 1984; McLaughlin and Weiss, 1991).

Intriguingly, activation of pro-MMP-1 is markedly increased in both speed and extent by the presence of MMP-3. This enzyme is capable of activating pro-MMP-1 on its own but the process is very slow. However, when pro-MMP-1 was treated with plasmin and subsequently with MMP-3 the activation was extremely rapid and the activity was greater than could be obtained by plasmin alone. It has been suggested that plasmin removes a portion of the pro-peptide of pro-MMP-1, which induces conformational changes rendering it readily susceptible to attack by MMP-3 (Suzuki *et al.*, 1990). The capability of MMP-3 to activate pro-MMP-1 suggests that activation of MMP-3 is a rate-limiting step in extracellular matrix degradation, particularly as MMP-3 can degrade other connective tissue components such as proteoglycans, fibronectin and laminin. In conditions of inflammation, plasma and tissue proteinases such as kallikrein and plasmin could accelerate the activation of pro-MMP-1 via MMP-3. This acceleration would of course be enhanced by the increased synthesis of these two enzymes through the influence of inflammatory mediators. However, since the angiogenic factor ESAF can also activate these pro-enzymes, the condition in which either of these mechanisms of activation occur or predominate needs to be studied.

Once the prometalloproteinases have been activated they are almost instantly inhibited by specific tissue inhibitors of metalloproteinases (TIMPs) (see p. 126). TIMP-1 binds non-covalently to active metalloproteinases in a 1:1 molar ratio and TIMP-1 can also form a complex with the pro-enzyme form of MMP-9. TIMP-2, a more recently isolated inhibitor, complexes specifically with the pro-enzyme form of MMP-2. These enzyme–inhibitor complexes, although non-covalently bound, have hitherto been considered to be irreversible, as it has not been possible to split them with proteolytic enzymes or with chemical activators of pro-enzymes. However, ESAF has been shown to be capable of splitting the enzyme–inhibitor complex and of releasing free active enzyme. In both instances, namely activation of pro-MMP-2 and reactivation of TIMP-1 and -2 inhibitor complexes, the amount of ESAF needed for the reactivation of enzyme–inhibitor complex and for activation of the pro-enzyme is in the picomolar range (McLaughlin and Weiss, 1991).

In the laboratory it is possible to activate all the pro-MMPs with organic mercurial compounds such as aminophenyl mercuric acetate (APMA) or mersalyl. These reagents are commonly used for laboratory studies in order to determine the quantity of pro-enzymes secreted by cells in culture. However, no organomercurial compound is able to reactivate the enzyme inhibitor complexes.

Synthesis of the MMPs by fixed tissue cells is greatly enhanced by some of the macrophage-derived inflammatory mediators such as interleukin 1 (IL-1) and tumour necrosis factor (TNF), also growth factors such as epidermal growth factor, platelet-derived growth factor (PDGF) and fibroblast growth factor. However, by contrast, transforming growth factorβ (TGFβ) inhibits MMP synthesis by other growth factors in cultured fibroblasts and induces the expression of TIMPs. This suggests that there is a switching-on process for the production of the MMPs and a controlling switching-off process which represses induction of the enzymes and simultaneously promotes *de novo* synthesis of the tissue inhibitors, thus ensuring removal of any excess enzyme.

Messenger RNAs for the MMPs can be induced by treatment with a variety of agents, such as cytokines, growth factors and tumour promoters. The mechanism by which growth factors induce the production of the MMPs is complex: however, it is now clear that the proto-oncogenes c-*fos* and c-*jun* play an important role in the regulation of metalloproteinase gene expression. This has been demonstrated using antisense RNA for c-*fos*, in which case induction of MMP-1 and MMP-3 gene expression was also inhibited. This seems to indicate that c-*fos* is needed for the stimulation of the messenger RNA for these metalloproteinases. Different growth factors stimulate either c-*fos* or c-*jun*. For example, PDGF appears to stimulate c-*fos* and TNFα c-*jun*. In contrast, TGFβ inhibits the synthesis of MMPs and recent evidence has shown that this inhibition also occurs at the level of transcription and probably involves c-*fos* or c-*jun*.

TISSUE INHIBITORS OF METALLOPROTEINASES

Human skin fibroblast TIMP-1 is a 28.5 kDa glycoprotein which inhibits the majority of the MMPs on a 1:1 molar stoichiometric basis via the formation of a very high affinity enzyme–inhibitor complex. Fibroblasts also secrete another inhibitor of the MMPs, namely TIMP-2. Both TIMPs contain 12 cysteine residues, all of which are thought to be involved in intramolecular disulphide bridges. TIMP-2 appears to be a specific inhibitor of MMP-2. As has been mentioned previously, TGFβ stimulates the production of TIMP-1 by human skin fibroblasts either alone or in conjunction with IL-1 (Wright et al., 1991). Not all fibroblast cell lines respond to these growth factors in the same manner: some cell lines respond to stimulation by both growth factors, others by TGFβ alone.

Note added in proof. The nomenclature of numbered MMPs has now been discarded in favour of interstitial collagenase for MMP-1 and neutrophil collagenase for MMP-8 gelatinase A and B for MMP-2 and -9 respectively, and stromelysin 1 and 2 for MMPs-3 and -10 respectively.

ELASTASE

Elastase is really a blanket term for a group of disparate types of enzymes capable of degrading either soluble elastin or a synthetic substrate, N-succinyl-(trialanine) p-nitroanilide. There is a considerable problem of nomenclature for the elastinolytic enzymes since fibroblast elastase has been classified by some workers as an intracellular metalloproteinase and by others as a serine proteinase. It is clear that much more work is required to unravel the problem, particularly for dermal fibroblasts.

The best-characterised elastases have been derived from polymorphonuclear cells and are generally known as neutrophil elastases. These are serine proteinases. Neutrophil elastase is present in the azurophil granules of the polymorphonuclear cells, and although it is termed an elastase it also cleaves the cross-linking regions of the fibrillar collagens, the helical region of types III and IV collagen, and it attacks fibronectin. Macrophage elastase is a metalloproteinase but like the neutrophil enzyme it is not specific. Pancreatic elastase, like the neutrophil enzyme, is a serine proteinase and both these proteinases hydrolyse peptide bonds in which a hydrophobic residue such as alanine, valine or leucine is the amino acid constituent.

An elastase-type enzyme has been isolated from vulval fibroblasts cultured from women suffering from lichen sclerosus et atrophicus. The enzyme was active against both insoluble elastin and the synthetic peptide trialanine p-nitroanilide. The enzyme was a metalloenzyme and may be responsible for the loss of elastic fibres reported in the superficial dermis of patients suffering from this disease (Godeau et al., 1982). Stimulation of elastase synthesis in human skin fibroblasts by IL-1 obtained from conditioned medium from cultured keratinocytes, and also by recombinant IL-1 has been reported (Croute *et al.*, 1991) and perhaps synthesis of the metalloenzyme is controlled in the same or a similar manner to that of MMPs.

REFERENCES

Bachinger HP, Morris NP, Lunstrum GP, Keene DR, Rosenbaum LM, Compton LA and Burgeson RE (1990) The relationship of the biophysical and biochemical characteristics of type VII collagen to the function of anchoring fibrils. *Journal of Biological Chemistry* **265**, 10095–10101.

Burgeson RE and Morris NP (1987) The collagen family of proteins. In: Uitto J and Perejda AJ (eds) *Connective Tissue Disease: Molecular Pathology of the Extracellular Matrix*, pp. 3–28. New York: Marcel Dekker.

Croute F, Delaporte E, Bonnefoy JY, Fertin C, Thivolet A and Nicholas SJF (1991) Interleukin-1 stimulates fibroblast elastase activity. *British Journal of Dermatology* **124**, 538–541.

Dahlback K, Ljungquist A, Lofberg H, Dahlback B, Engvall E and Sakai LY (1990) Fibrillin immunoreactive fibers constitute a unique network in the human dermis: immunohistochemical comparison of the distribution of fibrillin, vitronectin, amyloid P component and orcein stainable structures in the human skin. *Journal of Investigative Dermatology* **94**, 284–291.

Davies NR and Anwar RA (1970) On the mechanism of formation of desmosine and isodesmosine cross-links of elastin. *J Am Chem Soc* **92**, 3778.

Fleischmajer R, Jacobs L, Schwartz E and Sakai LY (1991) Elastin-associated microfibrils (10 nm) in a three-dimensional fibroblast culture. *Laboratory Investigation* **64**, 791.

Gibson MA, Hughes JL, Fanning JC and Cleary EG (1989) The major antigen of elastin-associated microfibrils is a 31-kDa glycoprotein. *Journal of Biological Chemistry* **261**, 11429–11436.

Godeau G, Frances C, Hornebeck W, Brechemier D and Robert L (1982) Isolation and partial characterisation of an elastase-type protease in human vulva fibroblasts: its possible involvement in vulvar elastic tissue destruction of patients with lichen sclerosus et atrophicus. *Journal of Investigative Dermatology* **78**, 270–275.

Holbrook KA and Byers PH (1987) Diseases of the extracellular matrix: structural alterations of collagen fibrils in skin. In: Uitto J and Perejda AJ (eds) *Connective Tissue Disease: Molecular Pathology of the Extracellular Matrix*, pp. 101–142. New York: Marcel Dekker.

Keene DR, Lundstrum GP, Morris NP, Stoddard DW and Burgeson RE (1991) Two type XII-like collagens localise to the surface of banded collagen fibrils. *Journal of Cell Biology* **113**, 971–978.

Kielty CM, Cummings C, Whittaker SP, Shuttleworth CA and Grant M (1991) Isolation and ultrastructural analysis of microfibrillar structures from foetal bovine elastic tissues: relative abundance and supramolecular architecture of type VI collagen assemblies and fibrillin. *Journal of Cell Science* **99**, 797–807.

Kivirikko K and Kuivaniemi H (1987) Post translational modifications of collagen and their alterations in heritable diseases. In: Uitto J and Perejda AJ (eds) *Connective Tissue Disease: Molecular Pathology of the Extracellular Matrix*, pp. 263–292. New York: Marcel Dekker.

Lee B, Godrey M, Vitale E, *et al.* (1991) Linkage of Marfan syndrome and a phenotypically related disorder to two different fibrillin genes. *Nature* **352**, 330–334.

Li K, Sawarmura D, Guidice GJ, Diaz LA, Mattei M-G, Chu M-L, Uitto J (1991) Genomic organisation of collagenous domains and chromosomal assignment of human 180-kDa bullous pemphigoid antigen-2, a novel vollagen of stratified squamous epithelium. *J Biol Chem* **266**, 24064–24069.

Maddox BK, Sakai LY, Keene DR and Glanville RW (1989) Connective tissue microfibrils: isolation and characterisation of 3 large pepsin resistant domains of fibrillin. *Journal of Biological Chemistry* **264**, 21381–21385.

McLaughlin B, Cawston T and Weiss JB (1991) Activation of the matrix metalloproteinase inhibitor complex by a low molecular weight angiogenic factor. *Biochimica et Biophysica Acta* **1073**, 295–298.

Matrisian L (1990) Metalloproteinases and their inhibitors in matrix remodelling. *Trends in Genetics* **6**, 121–125.

McLaughlin B and Weiss JB (1991) The proform of matrix metalloproteinase-2 is activated by endothelial cell stimulating angiogenesis factor. *Intnl J Microcirc* **10** (4), 401.

Okada Y, Morodomi T, Enghild JJ, Suzuki K, Yasui A, Nakanish I, Salvasen G and Nagasi H (1990) Matrix metalloproteinase 2 from human rheumatoid synovial fibroblasts: purification and activation of the precursor and enzymic properties. *European Journal of Biochemistry* **194**, 721–730.

Parente MG, Chung LC, Ryyanen J, Woodley DT, Wynn KC, Bauer EA, Mattei MG, Chu ML and Uitto J (1991) Human type VII collagen: cDNA cloning and chromosomal mapping of the gene. *Proceedings of the National Academy of Sciences USA* **88**, 6931–6935.

Ross R (1973) The elastic fiber. *Journal of Histochemistry and Cytochemistry* **21**(3), 199–208.

Suzuki K, Enghild JJ, Morodomi T, Salvasen G and Nagasi H (1990) Mechanisms of activation of tissue procollagenase by matrix metalloproteinase 3 (stromelysin). *Biochemistry* **29**, 10261–10269.

Uitto J and Perejda AJ (eds) (1987) *Connective Tissue Disease: Molecular Pathology of the Extra cellular Matrix*. New York: Marcel Dekker.

Van Der Rest M and Garrone R (1991) Collagen family of proteins. *FASEB Journal* **5**, 2814–2823.

Weiss JB, Elstow SF, Hill C, McLaughlin B, Schor A and Ayad S (1984) Low molecular weight angiogenesis factor: a growth factor not unique to tumours, which activates procollagenase. *Progress in Applied Microcirculation* (1984) **4**, 76–87.

Wright JK, Cawston TE and Hazleman BL (1991) Transforming growth factor β stimulates production of the tissue inhibitor of metalloproteinases by human synovial and skin fibroblasts.

RECOMMENDED FURTHER READING

Matrisian L (1992) Matrix degrading metalloproteinases. *Bioessays* **14**, 455–463.

Shaw LM and Olsen BR (1991) FACIT collagens: diverse molecular bridges in extracellular matrices. *Trends in Biochemical Science* **16**, 191–194.

Van Der Rest M and Garrone R (1991) Collagen family of proteins. *FASEB Journal* **5**, 2814–2823.

APPENDIX

Single-letter notation for amino acids used in this chapter:

Alanine, A; Arginine, R; Aspartic acid, D; Cysteine, C; Leucine, L; Lysine, K; Proline, P; Valine, V.

7 Cytokines

MICHAEL J. CORK, JOHN B. MEE and GORDON W. DUFF

Cell proliferation within the epidermis is normally tightly controlled so that the production of keratinocytes in the basal layer balances the loss from the horny layer. If the skin is injured an increased production of keratinocytes occurs. This proliferation can be achieved if quiescent (G_0) keratinocytes are triggered into the cell cycle and/or the cell cycle time is reduced, permitting more cell divisions within a set time (Wright and Alison, 1984). When the wound has been repaired, the kinetics of keratinocyte proliferation return to a resting state. A similar increase in the proportion of keratinocytes in cycle occurs in inflammatory dermatoses such as psoriasis, in which infiltrating immune cells interact with the resident keratinocytes, Langerhans cells, endothelial cells and fibroblasts. It now appears that the homeostatic control mechanism in the skin is a complex network of cytokines mediating interactions between these resident cells and T-lymphocytes, neutrophils and macrophages.

Cytokines can be defined as inducible, water-soluble, protein mediators of molecular weight greater than 5 kDa, which exert specific, receptor-mediated effects in target cells and/or the cytokine-producing cells themselves. Their biological functions involve the regulation of cell proliferation and function, but can be both stimulatory and inhibitory. Cytokines act in sets, and to understand their actions the biological context in which they act must be understood. For example, in a fibroblast cell line, transforming growth factor β (TGFβ) inhibits cell proliferation in the presence of epidermal growth factor (EGF), but stimulates proliferation in the presence of platelet-derived growth factor (PDGF). Each cytokine may be produced by many cells and in turn may exert an effect on many cell types. The cytokines bind to specific cell surface receptors which then produce a second message, for example via the protein kinase C or protein kinase A systems. Ultimately, the signal transduction pathway interacts with nuclear transcription factors such as c-*fos* and c-*jun*, which in turn regulate the transcription of particular genes and thereby produce a biological response (Fig. 7.1).

The terminology of peptide growth factors is confusing because different groups of scientists have used their own versions. Haematologists have identified colony stimulating factors, while immunologists have described lymphokines, cytokines and interleukins, and tumour biologists growth factors.

Molecular Aspects of Dermatology. Edited by G.C. Priestley.
© 1993 by John Wiley & Sons Ltd

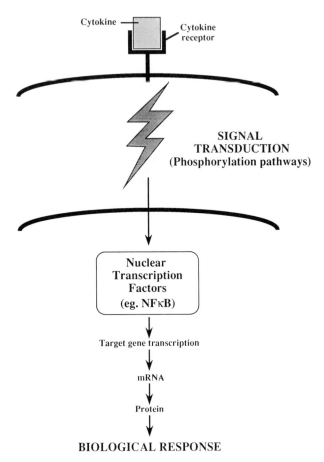

Fig. 7.1. Cellular activation pathway of cytokines

Table 7.1 lists the members of these different groups, although theoretically the term cytokine could cover them all and will be used here. The name ascribed to each cytokine is often based on the initial source or activity described for it, but as numerous activities and producer cells have subsequently been described for each cytokine these names have become less representative. This is exemplified by PDGF, which is produced by many other cells apart from platelets, including endothelial cells, smooth muscle cells and fibroblasts. For several cytokines, numerous factors with similar structure and activity have been described. For example endogenous pyrogen, haemopoietin 1, lymphocyte-activating factor and epidermal thymocyte activating factor are all interleukin 1 (IL-1). The cytokines can be regarded as the alphabet of a biological regulatory language, the text of which remains to be discovered (Sporn and Roberts, 1990).

Cytokines can act in an autocrine or paracrine mode, although they may also have systemic endocrine actions, for example keratinocyte-derived IL-1

Table 7.1. Cytokines, growth factors and colony-stimulating factors

Interleukins[a]	
IL-1α	Interleukin 1α
IL-1β	Interleukin 1β
IL-2 to IL-13	Interleukin 2 to interleukin 13
Interferons	
IFN-α	Interferon α
IFN-β	Interferon β
IFN-γ	Interferon γ
Cytotoxins	
TNFα	Tumour necrosis factor α
TNFβ	Tumour necrosis factor β
Colony-stimulating factors	
G-CSF	Granulocyte colony stimulating factor
M-CSF	Macrophage colony stimulating factor
GM-CSF	Granulocyte macrophage colony stimulating factor
SCF	Stem cell factor
Kit ligand	—
Multi-CSF (IL-3)	Multi-colony stimulating factor
Growth factors	
EGF	Epidermal growth factor
TGFα	Transforming growth factor α
TGFβ	Transforming growth factor β
aFGF	Acidic fibroblast growth factor
bFGF	Basic fibroblast growth factor
PDGF	Platelet-derived growth factor
BMP	Bone morphogenic protein

[a] Interleukins are defined as proteins which: (1) have a known amino acid sequence; (2) are produced by leukocytes (though not exclusively); and (3) are active in inflammation or immunity.

(Fig. 7.2). The autocrine and paracrine actions of cytokines provide a mechanism by which cells can communicate in their local micro-environment to produce integrated processes in all cells.

It is a basic principle that the biological response to a cytokine is a function of the balance between the production of the cytokine, the expression of its receptors on target cells and the presence of inhibitors. The isolated measurement of cytokine protein can therefore provide only limited physiological information and should always be accompanied by quantification of receptor expression and inhibitor levels.

CYTOKINES AND THE SKIN

Although virtually every cytokine may interact with the skin, there are several which have a central role in the regulation of cell proliferation, differentiation and function within it.

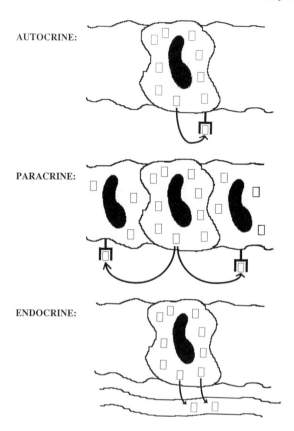

AUTOCRINE:

PARACRINE:

ENDOCRINE:

Fig. 7.2. Mechanisms of action of keratinocyte-derived IL-1

INTERLEUKIN 1

There are two classes of IL-1 molecule – IL-1α and IL-1β – each encoded by a separate gene on chromosome 2, but they seem to act on common receptors. IL-1 and tumour necrosis factor α (TNFα) are primary cytokines, which can stimulate their own production and the production of a large number of secondary cytokines (Fig. 7.3). The cells of the mononuclear phagocyte lineage are a major source of IL-1 and the released form is predominantly IL-1β (di Giovine and Duff, 1990). The wide range of biological actions of IL-1 seems to be involved in the control of immune and inflammatory responses by induction of lymphocytotropic cytokines involved in the proliferation and differentiation of B- and T-cells (e.g. IL-1 itself, IL-2, IL-3, IL-4, IL-5, IL-6, IL-7, IL-8, TNFα, TNFβ, granulocyte–macrophage colony-stimulating factor (GM-CSF), and IL-2 receptor (IL-2R) and by the activation of vascular endothelial cells and connective tissue cells.

There are two forms of IL-1 receptor – types 1 and 2 (IL-1R1, IL-1R2) – which differ in their binding affinities, signal transduction and cell surface expression. Transformed T-cells and fibroblasts express IL-1R1, while neutrophils and B-cells express IL-1R2. IL-1 stimulates biological responses at very low levels of receptor occupancy. Only three to seven receptors per cell need to be occupied to produce a maximal response.

Pro-inflammatory cytokines are part of the innate immune response that combats infection and promotes wound healing, but if their actions are not controlled they can themselves cause extensive tissue damage and the death of the host. Two groups of inhibitors appear to be central to the physiological control of IL-1 and other cytokines. Type I inhibitor proteins are structural homologues of a cytokine that compete with it for binding to its receptor, e.g. the IL-1 receptor antagonist (IL-1ra). Binding of the IL-1ra to the IL-1 receptor does not produce detectable cell activation and so IL-1ra acts as a competitive inhibitor. The IL-1ra gene is located on chromosome 2 in the same region as IL-1α and IL-1β, and this organisation may be associated with coordinate regulation. Type II inhibitor proteins are soluble receptors, shed from the cell surface, which can bind a cytokine extracellularly and so prevent binding to receptors on target cells.

IL-1 in the skin

The epidermis contains levels of IL-1 that are 100–1000 times greater than those in most normal tissues. Keratinocytes are the major source of IL-1 in the epidermis and, unlike monocytes, are able to produce it constitutively without extrinsic stimulation (Kupper et al., 1986), though it is difficult to exclude inadvertent stimulation during cell processing (e.g. by bacterial endotoxin or ultraviolet (UV) light). The sequestration of IL-1 inside keratinocytes is a powerful protective mechanism against trauma and other stimuli, which by releasing a large pre-formed pool of IL-1 can trigger a rapid inflammatory response.

Keratinocytes in normal epidermis express only a few high-affinity receptors for IL-1, but this is increased in response to UVB radiation and trauma. IL-1 receptors can also be induced on keratinocytes by T-cell-derived interferon γ (IFNγ). The inducibility of IL-1 receptors on keratinocytes in the presence of static levels of IL-1 may be very important for the regulation of immune and inflammatory responses in the skin (Kupper, 1990).

A specific epithelial form of the IL-1ra has been cloned from lysates of keratinocytes and appears to be predominantly intracellular (icIL-1ra) (Haskill et al., 1991). The production of icIL-1ra by cultured keratinocytes is increased in culture conditions which promote their differentiation. This is in contrast to the production of IL-1α by keratinocytes in culture, which decreases as they differentiate. Keratinocyte icIL-1ra may be important in the control of inflammation triggered by IL-1α released from dead or damaged keratinocytes and those primed to release IL-1 by other mechanisms, e.g. T-cell-derived IFNγ. Dysregulation of the production and release of icIL-1ra could contribute to a loss of IL-1 homeostasis and the development of inflammatory dermatoses.

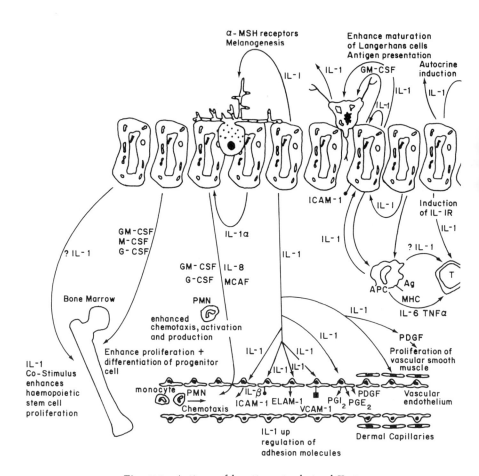

Fig. 7.3. Actions of keratinocyte-derived IL-1

Keratinocytes in normal skin can be considered to be in a 'resting state' (Kupper, 1990) (Fig. 7.4). IL-1 is sequestered within them and there are also high levels of the icIL-1ra and low expression of the IL-1 receptors. If keratinocytes are traumatised by physical injury or UV radiation, IL-1α is released and can activate keratinocytes by autocrine and paracrine mechanisms to produce secondary cytokines such as GM-CSF, IL-8, IL-6, M-CSF, G-CSF and further IL-1. These cytokines then initiate the production of an inflammatory infiltrate and activate fibroblasts to proliferate and produce collagen for wound healing. T-cell derived IFNγ induces expression of IL-1 receptors, which increases the biological effect of the IL-1 released from the keratinocytes. IL-1 released from keratinocytes has effects on many dermal and

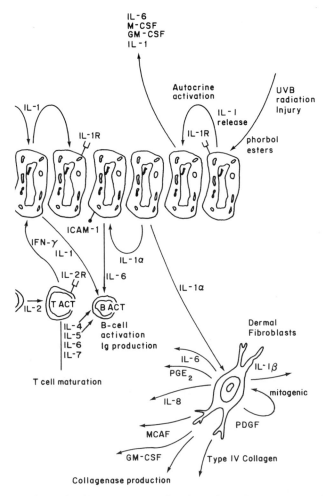

epidermal cells (Fig. 7.3) and is thought to have a pivotal role in the initiation of the local and systemic inflammatory responses (Cork and Duff, 1993).

In normal epidermis, IL-1 is intracellular. Its actions therefore depend on stimuli that induce its release and the expression of its receptor. The production of GM-CSF and IL-6 by keratinocytes is related to the number of IL-1 receptors which they are expressing. IFNγ is a potent stimulator of keratinocyte IL-1 receptor expression (Kupper *et al.*, 1986) and is released by activated T-cells in psoriasis. Thus T-cells can up-regulate IL-1 receptors on keratinocytes via IFNγ and so permit their activation by IL-1 and other pro-inflammatory cytokines.

IL-1 in psoriasis

The importance of investigating the production of a cytokine in relation to its receptors and inhibitors is illustrated by the dysregulation of IL-1 in psoriasis.

Resting keratinocyte   Activated keratinocyte

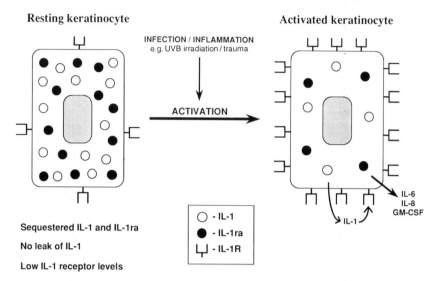

Sequestered IL-1 and IL-1ra

No leak of IL-1

Low IL-1 receptor levels

Fig. 7.4. Hypothetical model of keratinocyte activation

The levels of IL-1α are *reduced* in psoriatic lesional skin compared to normal skin (Gearing *et al.*, 1990), yet the production of secondary cytokines such as IL-8 and IL-6 is considerably *increased* in psoriatic lesional skin. These observations can be explained by the results of sequential biopsies of psoriatic non-lesional skin as it becomes lesional. IL-1α decreases into the lesion, but the IL-1 receptor antagonist also decreases and the IL-1 receptors increase considerably into the lesion (Mee *et al.*, 1992). The biological response to IL-1 is therefore considerably enhanced, permitting the production of secondary cytokines such as IL-8.

INTERLEUKIN 2

IL-2 is released by T-helper cells in association with MHC antigens and bound IL-1. IL-2 promotes the clonal expansion of T-cells and induces the expression of the IL-2 receptor. One of the components of this receptor, the soluble α chain or tac protein (sIL-2R), is shed from the T-cell membrane in proportion to the degree of T-cell activation. Circulating levels of the sIL-2R are elevated in patients with atopic eczema and psoriasis (Colver *et al.*, 1989; Kemmett *et al.*, 1989).

IL-2 also induces the production of other cytokines by T-cells, including interferons, IL-4, IL-5, IL-7 and GM-CSF (Luger *et al.*, 1989). IFNγ stimulates keratinocytes to express IL-1 receptors and to produce TGFα, which can stimulate their proliferation. The importance of the activated T-cell in inflammatory dermatoses is illustrated by the action of cyclosporin A, which inhibits the release of IL-2 from T-cells and the production of its receptors, and can provide good control of severe atopic eczema and psoriasis.

TUMOUR NECROSIS FACTOR α

TNFα, also known as cachectin, was initially isolated as a factor producing haemorrhagic necrosis of tumours, but has subsequently been shown to have a wide range of effects on immune and connective tissue cells (Patton et al., 1989). TNFα activates lymphocytes, neutrophils, eosinophils, macrophages and osteoclasts. TNFα exerts a range of biological responses depending on the concentration produced. At low concentrations it induces tissue remodelling, stimulating the growth of fibroblasts and increasing production of collagenase. At intermediate concentrations it has a protective role in combating infection, increasing neutrophil and monocyte chemotaxis, stimulating phagocytosis and enhancing superoxide production. The protective effect of TNFα is illustrated by its protective action against parasites such as toxoplasma, leishmania and schistosomes. At very high concentrations TNFα produces the potentially fatal manifestations of septic shock.

TNFα affects tumour cells by a direct cytotoxic action and induces necrosis by damaging the tumour vasculature. It has many actions similar to IL-1: they can both stimulate the production of each other and TNFα can stimulate its own production and that of secondary cytokines such as IL-6, IL-8, GM-CSF, M-CSF, PDGF and TGFβ.

TNFα in the epidermis

TNFα is one of the cytokines produced by activated keratinocytes (Table 7.2), its production being increased by UVB radiation and endotoxin. TNFα secreted by keratinocytes and dermal macrophages may contribute to the induction of signs of skin inflammation such as ulceration. It also has a spectrum of divergent actions in the skin, from beneficial to toxic. TNFα together with IL-1 and GM-CSF may function as an essential signal for Langerhans cell viability within the epidermis (Koch et al., 1990). TNFα may promote wound healing by stimulating the growth of fibroblasts and remodelling the extracellular matrix.

The role of TNFα in the aetiology of inflammatory dermatoses, connective tissue diseases and other autoimmune diseases is also divergent. It enhances the immune response by inducing the expression of HLA-DR and adhesion molecules ICAM-1 (intercellular adhesion molecule 1) and ELAM on keratinocytes and fibroblasts. This permits the binding of T-cells, neutrophils and other immune cells. Dermal dendrocytes producing TNFα have been demonstrated in the papillae of psoriatic lesions. Monocytes from psoriatic lesions produce increased levels of TNFα and GM-CSF (Pigatto et al., 1989), which may stimulate neutrophils directly and activate keratinocytes to release further cytokines such as IL-8. TNFα may cause the cutaneous manifestations of graft-versus-host disease directly, as these changes are prevented by anti-TNFα antibodies in mice.

In contrast, in NZB mice, which develop a disease like systemic lupus, low

Table 7.2. Keratinocyte-derived cytokines and related molecules

Interleukins	Growth factors	Colony-stimulating factors
IL-1α	EGF	G-CSF
IL-1β	TGFα	M-CSF
IL-1R(I)	TGFβ	GM-CSF
IL-1R(II)	bFGF	
IL-1ra	PDGF AA	
IL-3	PDGF B	
IL-6	TNFα	
IL-8		

levels of TNFα have been demonstrated, and pretreatment of the mice with TNFα delays the onset of lupus nephritis (Jacob and McDevitt, 1988). The onset of diabetes mellitus in non-obese mice can also be prevented by the injection of TNFα (Jacob *et al.*, 1991). These observations imply that in some circumstances TNFα may have a protective effect against the development of auto-immune disease.

TUMOUR NECROSIS FACTOR β

TNFβ and TNFα have overlapping functions and bind to the same receptors. TNFβ is a mediator of killing by cytotoxic T-cells, natural killer (NK) cells and lymphokine-activated killer cells. It is produced by these cells after exposure to antigen in the context of MHC or by high levels of IL-2. TNFβ may be a central mediator of the defence against viruses, particularly in the destruction of virally infected cells.

TNFβ has also been implicated in the development of some auto-immune diseases such as diabetes mellitus, multiple sclerosis and scleroderma/polymyositis overlap. The production of soluble forms of the TNF receptors may provide a new therapeutic approach to these diseases.

EPIDERMAL GROWTH FACTOR

Epidemal growth factor (EGF) is produced by multiple cell types and stimulates epidermal growth and differentiation directly (Carpenter and Cohen, 1979). The physiological role of EGF has been difficult to establish because of its multiple origins and ability to stimulate the growth of many cell types. The receptor for EGF is expressed on many cell types, including mesenchymal and epithelial cells.

EGF stimulates the growth and migration of keratinocytes in culture. In normal human epidermis, EGF receptors are present in highest concentration in the basal layer and decrease in the differentiating keratinocytes as they move up through the epidermis. In contrast, in psoriatic lesions EGF receptors are present in all layers of the epidermis (Nanney *et al.*, 1986). Uninvolved psoriatic epidermis also shows increased expression of EGF receptors within the horny and spinous layers). EGF also stimulates dermal fibroblast proliferation and collagen production *in vitro*.

TRANSFORMING GROWTH FACTOR α

Transforming growth factor α (TGFα) was originally named because of its ability to induce anchorage-independent growth (a characteristic of trans-formed cells) in rat kidney cells in culture (Derynck, 1988). A third of the amino acids of TGFα are homologous with those of EGF and it binds to the EGF receptor. TGFα acts as a mitogenic agent for EGF-responsive cells, i.e. keratinocytes, fibroblasts and endothelial cells, regulating both the growth and differentiation of keratinocytes (Coffey *et al.*, 1988). TGFα is more potent than EGF in inducing keratinocyte colony expansion and has a much greater affinity for the EGF receptor than EGF itself.

TGFα is present in normal epidermis but its levels are elevated in psoriatic plaques (Elder *et al.*, 1989). TGFα mRNA is localised in high-level keratinocytes in psoriatic plaques, indicating that it is produced by keratinocytes rather than dermal macrophages. Experiments using transgenic mice that are hyper-producers of TGFα indicate that although TGFα may cause keratinocyte hyperproliferation, it is not a primary initiating cytokine in psoriasis.

TRANSFORMING GROWTH FACTOR β

Transforming growth factor β (TGFβ) is structurally distinct from TGFα and exists in at least four dimeric forms. It has been isolated from fibroblasts, endothelial cells, monocytes and keratinocytes and binds to a specific receptor (Barnard *et al.*, 1988). TGFβ inhibits keratinocyte proliferation but stimulates fibroblast growth and the formation of extracellular matrix. TGFβ may have a central role in the degradation and remodelling of the extracellular matrix which is crucial for those cell-to-cell interactions that regulate proliferation and differentiation (Sporn and Roberts, 1990).

It has been postulated that a deficiency of TGFβ could explain the epidermal hyperproliferation in psoriasis, but Elder *et al.* (1989) found no significant difference in TGFβ mRNA levels between normal and psoriatic uninvolved and lesional epidermis.

INTERLEUKIN 4

Interleukin 4 (IL-4) is a 20 kDa polypeptide which is normally produced by CD4 + T-lymphocytes and cells of the mast cell lineage. The IL-4 gene is located on the long arm of chromosome 5 in the close proximity to the genes for IL-5, GM-CSF, IL-3, IL-9, M-CSF and other cytokine-related genes (Thompson, 1992).

IL-4 acts at several levels of antigen-independent B-cell development and antigen-dependent B-cell activation, proliferation and differentiation. B-lymphocytes are induced to increase expression of MHC class II molecules and the low-affinity IgE receptor CD23. IL-4 causes switching of lipopolysaccharide (LPS)-activated B-cells to IgE and IgG1 production.

It is now established that two sets of immunoregulatory CD4+ T-cells influence the outcome of infection. TH1 cells produce IL-2 and IFNγ and preferentially activate macrophages to kill or inhibit the growth of a pathogen, resulting in mild, self-limiting disease. In contrast, T-cells producing IL-4 and IL-5 are termed TH2 cells. They augment humoral responses and inhibit some cell-mediated responses, resulting in fulminant infection.

IL-4 inhibits the production of IL-1, but increases the production of the IL-1 receptor antagonist (Vannier *et al.*, 1992). IL-4 therefore not only reduces the production of IL-1 but further reduces the biological response by increasing the production of its inhibitor IL-1ra. IL-4 also suppresses the production of IL-6, IL-8 and TNFα, providing another mechanism to further reduce the inflammatory response to bacterial and viral infections.

The pattern of cytokine response to an infection can determine the clinical pattern and outcome. For example, in patients infected with *Mycobacterium leprae*, a predominant TH1 cell response produces resistance to *M. leprae* and tuberculoid leprosy. In contrast, the TH2 cytokines IL-4, IL-5 and IL-10 predominate in the lesions of patients with widespread lepromatous disease. The IFNγ was derived from CD4+ T-cells, while the IL-4 was produced by CD8+ T-suppressor cells. Furthermore, the fatal outcome of *Leishmania major* infection in mice correlates with a T-cell response which predominantly produces IL-4.

In atopic eczema CD4+ T-cells are the major infiltrating cell type in eczematous lesions. When these cells are extracted, they are found to produce high levels of IL-4 and low levels of IFNγ in response to house dust-mite antigen (*Dermatophagoides pteronyssinus*). These observations led to uncontrolled clinical trials of IFNγ in severe atopic eczema. Some patients responded to this treatment clinically with a corresponding fall in serum IgE levels and IgE production *in vitro*.

The production of transgenic mice has further enhanced our understanding of the role of IL-4 *in vivo*. In mice homozygous for a mutation which inactivates the IL-4 gene, the serum levels of IgE and IgG1 were markedly reduced and no IgE response to a nematode infection occurred (Kuhn *et al.*, 1991). The opposite picture occurs in transgenic mice in which the IL-4 gene has been fused to an immunoglobulin enhancer/promoter. The over-expression of IL-4 results in very high IgE levels and an increase in the population of CD8+ T-cells (Tepper *et al.*, 1990) These mice also developed an allergic blepharitis.

Increased production of IL-4 therefore has a central role in the production of allergic inflammatory dermatoses such as atopic eczema. IL-4 also attenuates (with IL-5 and IL-10) the immune response to pathogens such as *M. leprae* and

Leishmania, leading to fulminant infection. Dysregulation of the IL-4 gene may therefore be central to the development of these diseases.

INTERLEUKIN 6

Interleukin 6 (IL-6), like IL-1, is a ubiquitous pro-inflammatory cytokine, which is released immediately after injury (Thompson, 1992). It was initially termed B-cell activating factor 2 because of its ability to induce antibody secretion by pre-activated B-cells. IL-6 is produced by monocytes, T-cells, fibroblasts, endothelial cells and keratinocytes. Its production is increased by other cytokines such as TNFα, IL-1, interferons, PDGF and bacterial toxins (Luger *et al.*, 1989). IL-6 is a major mediator of the acute-phase response and is an endogenous pyrogen. In addition to enhancement of B-cell growth and differentiation, IL-6 augments early events in T-cell activation and can'function as a second signal for T-cell proliferation.

IL-6 may be involved in the pathogenesis of certain autoimmune diseases. Very high levels of IL-6 have been detected in the synovial fluid of patients with rheumatoid arthritis but not in those with active osteoarthritis. Excessive production of IL-6 may induce polyclonal B-cell activation, resulting in hypergammaglobulinaemia and antibody production. This occurs in patients with myeloma, plasmacytoma, atrial myxoma and Castleman's disease, which is characterised by a benign hyperplastic lymphadenopathy associated with fever, increased immunoglobulin levels and, occasionally, skin lesions.

IL-6 is another cytokine produced by activated keratinocytes (Table 7.2). Its production is increased in keratinocytes from psoriatic lesions and it stimulates the proliferation of keratinocytes *in vitro*. These observations led to speculation that IL-6 may have a primary initiating role in psoriasis, although recent observations in transgenic mice which selectively over-express IL-6 have not supported this idea. There was no enhanced epidermal proliferation, abnormal differentiation or inflammation. The only abnormality in these mice was thickening of the horny layer (Turksen *et al.*, 1992).

INTERLEUKIN 8

Interleukin 8 (IL-8) is a member of a superfamily of host defence and chemotactic cytokines with similar structures (Schroder, 1992). One subfamily has preferential chemotactic activity for neutrophils (IL-8). The other subfamily has chemotactic activity for other leukocytes, e.g. monocyte chemotactic and activating factor (MCAF).

IL-8 is produced by monocytes, T-cells, endothelial cells, dermal fibroblasts, keratinocytes and neutrophils themselves. Keratinocytes do not produce IL-8 constitutively but this is stimulated by other cytokines, e.g. IL-1α, IL-1β and TNFα. The addition of IFNγ to TNFα significantly enhances the production of IL-8.

Neutrophils are a significant part of the inflammatory infiltrate in psoriatic lesions, and large amounts of IL-8 have been isolated from psoriatic scales (Gearing *et al.*, 1990). Sequential biopsies across the edge of an enlarging psoriatic plaque demonstrate low levels of IL-8 outside the plaque but very high levels within it (Mee *et al.*, 1992). It is probable that IL-8 is released from keratinocytes following activation by IL-1.

INTERLEUKIN 10

IL-10 is a 35–40 kDa protein which is produced by the TH0 and TH2 subsets of helper T-cells. IL-10 was initially termed cytokine synthesis inhibitory factor because of its ability to inhibit the production of other cytokines by TH1 T-cells (Zlotnik and Moore, 1991). IL-10 inhibits the production of all cytokines produced by TH1 T-cells (e.g. IL-2, TNFβ and IFNγ), but the inhibition of IFNγ production is maximal. IL-10 may therefore be important in suppressing delayed hypersensitivity reactions and other TH1 cell-mediated responses. IL-10 also inhibits the production of IL-8, IL-1α, IL-6, GM-CSF, G-CSF and TNFα by monocytes/macrophages and decreases their expression of MHC class II molecules. Although IL-10 inhibits many T-cell functions, it stimulates the proliferation and differentiation of B-cells into antibody-secreting plasma cells.

Comparison of the sequence information for IL-10 with part of the protein-coding region of the Epstein–Barr virus genome revealed very close sequence homology. There is more than 80% homology between the amino acid sequence of IL-10 and BCRF1 (B-cell regulatory factor 1/vIL-10). Only a subset of the activities of IL-10 has been conserved by vIL-10, e.g. the B-cell viability-enhancing activities which are manifest as the immortalisation of B-cells that have been transformed by the virus. BCRF1/vIL-10 may also inhibit T-cell and NK cell responses that would otherwise be activated in the early phase of infection by Epstein–Barr virus. Exploitation by viruses of captured genes encoding cytokines, their receptors, or other immunoregulatory molecules may be a mechanism to enable them to overcome the host defences.

The ability of IL-10 to suppress the production of cytokines including IL-2, IFNγ and IL-1α and up-regulate the production of the IL-1 receptor antagonist suggests that it could have a role in the treatment of inflammatory dermatoses such as psoriasis. Antagonism of the actions of IL-10 may have a role in the treatment of Epstein–Barr virus infection, e.g. cutaneous T-cell lymphoma.

COLONY-STIMULATING FACTORS

There are four major species of haemopoietic colony-stimulating factors: multilineage colony stimulating factor (interleukin 3, IL-3), granulocyte–macrophage colony stimulating factor (GM-CSF), macrophage colony stimulating factor (M-CSF) and granulocyte colony stimulating factor (G-CSF). These factors control the proliferation and differentiation of the haemopoietic stem cells, progenitor cells and their progency (Sporn and Roberts, 1990). Their action leads to an increased production of mature haemopoietic cells such as neutrophils, monocytes, eosinophils and erythrocytes.

The colony-stimulating factors are produced by many different cell types, following activation by endotoxins or other cytokines. TNFα, IL-1 and interferons stimulate GM-CSF production by monocytes, endothelial cells and fibroblasts. T-cells produce high levels of both GM-CSF and IL-3, and this is increased following stimulation with IL-2. Keratinocytes produce IL-3 and GM-CSF, and this is increased by UV radiation and by cytokines such as IL-1, TNFα, IL-4 and GM-CSF itself. Colony-stimulating factors therefore cause increased production of immunologically competent cells in response to cytokines released from keratinocytes, fibroblasts, endothelial cells, Langerhans cells and monocytes themselves, and produce a link between the epidermis, dermis, immune and haemopoietic systems.

High levels of GM-CSF have been demonstrated in lesional psoriatic skin and psoriatic scale. Monocytes from psoriatic skin enhance neutrophil function by producing GM-CSF. Neutrophils may enhance auto-immune skin diseases by adhering to anti-basement membrane antibodies, and this is markedly enhanced by GM-CSF. GM-CSF may therefore amplify the inflammatory response locally in psoriatic lesions by enhancing neutrophil adherence and function and increasing their production within the bone marrow.

REGULATION OF CYTOKINE GENE EXPRESSION

The primary cytokines IL-1α, IL-1β and TNFα are regarded as central regulators of inflammation, immunity and tissue remodelling. They have been implicated widely as mediators of skin and connective tissue diseases such as psoriasis, scleroderma, systemic lupus erythematosus and acne. Despite this, we have little information on how IL-1 and TNF genes are controlled in normal circumstances and even less on the mechanisms that might operate to increase gene expression in inflammatory dermatoses. It seems that, as with other cytokines, major transcriptional control is exerted on the IL-1s and TNF. Post-transcriptional mechanisms seem important too, particularly in the case of TNFα, where mRNA stability is markedly influenced by elements in the 3' untranslated regions.

It is known that accumulation rates of IL-1α, IL-1β and TNFα proteins show stable differences among individuals but it is unclear whether producer phenotype is related to transcriptional and/or post-transcriptional activities. If the former, then one mechanism could be the presence of polymorphisms within promoter or enhancer elements in the 5' flanking portion of genes. In both IL-1α and IL-1β it has been possible to identify stretches of 100–200 base pairs with dramatic enhancer properties and others with potent silencing properties. At least one of the sequence polymorphisms in the IL-1β gene occurs within such a stretch (Zhang and Duff, 1992). Several such areas contain viral response sequences.

Enhancer or suppressor sequences may also occur outside the 5' region. In IL-1α, for example, a restriction fragment length polymorphism maps to intron 6 and the variable length can be accounted for by different numbers of a 46 bp tandem repeat. Of interest is that each repeat contains a recognition sequence for the SP1 transcription factor, an imperfect viral enhancer element, and a glucocorticoid receptor binding site. Whether this polymorphism is reflected in differentially regulated gene expression or differential responses to glucocorticoids remains to be tested (Bailly *et al.*, 1993).

The first polymorphism within the human TNFX locus has recently been described (Wilson *et al.*, 1993). It is biallelic, lies within the promoter region, and the uncommon allele shows a very strong association with HLA A1, B8 and DR3 alleles, a haplotype known to have many autoimmune associations.

A five-allele polymorphism within intron 2 of the IL-1 receptor antagonist gene has been demonstrated. The alleles correspond to variable numbers of an 86 bp sequence, and Mendelian segregation of the alleles through three generations has been observed (Tarlow *et al.*, 1993). The number of repeats may be of functional significance as the sequence contains three potential protein binding sites which can regulate gene expression.

The frequency of the different alleles of each of these polymorphisms is being studied in the normal population and compared with that from inflammatory diseases such as psoriasis and systemic lupus erythematosus. Our working hypothesis is that allelic polymorphisms in genes that encode cytokines, their receptors and inhibitors contribute to the genetic basis of chronic inflammation. Genetic polymorphisms may be related to cytokine producer phenotypes and thus represent susceptibility and/or severity factors for chronic inflammatory diseases such as psoriasis. Increased or inappropriate expression of the genes for pro-inflammatory cytokines and associated molecules or decreased expression of genes for cytokines that inhibit pro-inflammatory cytokines (e.g. IL-4 and IL-10) are the possible consequences of polymorphisms in the regulatory sequences of such genes. This is now the most exciting area of cytokine research and has enormous therapeutic potential.

REFERENCES

Bailly S, di Giovine FS, Blakemore AIF and Duff GW (1993) Genetic polymorphism of interleukin-1α due to a variable number of intronic repeats. *European Journal of Immunology* (in press).
Barnard JA, Bascom CC, Lyons RM, Spies NJ and Moses HL (1988) Transforming growth factors in the control of epidermal proliferation. *American Journal of the Medical Sciences* **296**, 159–163.

Carpenter G and Cohen S (1979) Epidermal growth factor. *Annual Review of Biochemistry* **48**, 193–216.
Coffey RJ, Spies NJ, Bacon CC, Graves-Deal R, Pennington CY, Weissman BE and Moses HL (1988) Growth modulation of mouse keratinocytes by transforming growth factor alpha. *Cancer Research* **48**, 1596–1602.
Colver GB, Symons JA and Duff GW (1989) Soluble interleukin 2 receptor in atopic eczema. *British Medical Journal* **298**, 1426–1428.
Cork MJ and Duff GW (1993) Interleukin one. In: Luger TA and Schwartz T (eds) *Epidermal Cytokines and Growth Factors*. New York: Marcel Dekker (in press).
Derynck R (1988) Transforming growth factor α. *Cell* **54**, 593–595.
di Giovine FS and Duff GW (1990) Interleukin 1: the first interleukin. *Immunology Today* **11**, 13–20.
Elder JT, Fisher GJ, Lindquist PB, Bennett GL, Pittelkow MR, Coffey RJ, Ellingsworth L, Derynck R and Voorhees JJ (1989) Overexpression of transforming growth factor alpha in psoriatic epidermis. *Science* **243**, 811–814.
Gearing AJH, Fincham NJ, Bird CR, Wadhwa M, Meager A, Cartwright JE and Camp RDR (1990) Cytokines in skin lesions of psoriasis. *Cytokine* **2**, 68–75.
Haskill S, Martin G, Van Le L, Morris J, Peace A, Bigler CF, Jaffe GJ, Hammerberg C, Sporn SA, Fong S, Arend WP and Ralph P (1991) cDNA cloning of an intracellular form of the human interleukin 1 receptor antagonist associated with epithelium. *Proceedings of the National Academy of Sciences USA* **88**, 3681–3685.
Jacob CO and McDevitt HO (1988) Tumour necrosis factor-alpha in murine autoimmune 'lupus' nephritis. *Nature* **331**, 356–358.
Jacob CO, Hwang P, Lewis GD and Stall AM (1991) Tumour necrosis factor-alpha in murine systemic lupus erythematosus disease models: implications for genetic predisposition and immune reaction. *Cytokine* **3**, 551–561.
Kemmett D, Symons JA, Colver GB and Duff GW (1989) Serum-soluble interleukin-2 receptor in psoriasis: failure to reflect clinical improvement. *Acta Dermato-venereologica* **70**, 264–266.
Koch F, Heufler C, Kampgen E, Schneeweiss D, Bock G and Schuler G (1990) Tumour necrosis factor-alpha maintains viability of murine epidermal Langerhans cells in culture but in contrast to GM-CSF without inducing functional maturation. *Journal of Experimental Medicine* **171**, 159–171.
Kuhn R, Rajewsky K and Muller W (1991) Generation and analysis of interleukin-4 deficient mice. *Science* **254**, 707–709.
Kupper TS (1990) Role of epidermal cytokines. In: Oppenheim JJ and Sherach EM (eds) *Immunophysiology: The Role of Cells and Cytokines in Immunity and Inflammation*. Oxford: Oxford University Press.
Kupper TS, Ballard DW, Chua AO, McGuire JS, Flood PM, Horowitz MC, Langdon R, Lightfoot L and Gubler U (1986) Human keratinocytes contain mRNA indistinguishable from monocyte interleukin I alpha and beta mRNA. *Journal of Experimental Medicine* **164**, 2095–2100.
Luger TA, Schwarz T, Krutmann J, Kirnbauer R, Neuner P, Kock A, Urbanski A, Borth W and Schuer E (1989) Interleukin-6 is produced by epidermal cells and plays an important role in the activation of human T-lymphocytes and natural killer cells. *Annals of the New York Academy of Sciences* **557**, 405–414.
Mee JB, Cork MJ, di Giovine FS, blakemore AIF, Tarlow JK and Duff GW (1992) Induction pathway of cytokine gene expression across the advancing edge of psoriatic plaques. Proceedings of the 8th World Congress of Immunology, Budapest (abstract).
Nanney LB, Stoscheck CM, Magid M and King LE (1986) Altered ^{125}I epidermal growth factor binding and receptor distribution in psoriasis. *Journal of Investigative Dermatology* **86**, 260–265.

Patton JS, Rice GC, Ranges GE and Palladinoa MA (1989). In: Sorg CD (ed.) *Macrophage-derived Cell Regulatory Factors. Cytokines*, Vol. 1, p. 89. Basel: Karger.
Pigatto PD, Bersani L and Altonare G (1989) Presence of TNF and GM-CSF in secretion from untreated psoriatic monocyte. *Journal of Investigative Dermatology* **92**, 500 (abstract).
Schroder JM (1992) Chemotactic cytokines in the epidermis. *Experimental Dermatology* **1**, 12–19.
Sporn MB and Roberts AB (1990) *Peptide Growth Factors and their Receptors*, Vols 1 and 2. Berlin: Springer-Verlag.
Tarlow JK, Blakemore AIF, Lennard A, Solari R, Hughes HN, Steinkasserer A and Duff GW (1993) Polymorphism in human IL-1 receptor antagonist gene intron 2 is due to variable number of an 86 bp tandem repeat. *Human Genetics* (in press).
Tepper RI, Levinson DA, Stanger BZ, Camapos-Torres J, Abbas AK and Leder P (1990) IL-4 induces allergic-like inflammatory disease and alters T cell development in transgenic mice. *Cell* **62**, 457–467.
Thompson A (ed.) (1992) *The Cytokine Handbook*. London: Academic Press.
Turksen K, Kupper T, Degenstien L, Williams I and Fuchs E (1992) Interleukin 6: insights into its function in skin by overexpression in transgenic mice. *Proceedings of the National Academy of Sciences USA* **89**, 5068–5072.
Vannier E, Miller LC and Dinarello CA (1992) Coordinated anti-inflammatory effects of interleukin 4: interleukin 4 suppresses interleukin 1 production but upregulates gene expression and synthesis of interleukin 1 receptor antagonist. *Proceedings of the National Academy of Sciences USA* **89**, 4076–4080.
Wilson AG, de Vries N, Pociot F, van de Putte LBA and Duff GW (1992) An allelic polymorphism within the human tumour necrosis factor alpha (TNF-α) promoter region is strongly associated with HLA DR3. *Journal of Experimental Medicine* (in press).
Wright N and Alison M (1984) *The Biology of Epithelial Cell Populations*. Oxford: Clarendon Press.
Zhang G and Duff GW (1992) Regulation of the interleukin 1β gene. Proceedings of the 8th World Congress of Immunology, Budapest (abstract).
Zlotnik A and Moore KW (1991) Interleukin 10. *Cytokine* **3**, 366–371.

FURTHER READING

di Giovine FS, Stones S, Wojtacha D and Duff GW (1992) Cytokines: identification and measurement of gene activation. In: Gallacher G, Rees RC and Reynolds CW (eds) *Tumour Immunobiology: A Practical Approach*. Oxford: IRL Press.
Luger TA and Schwarz T (1992) *Epidermal Cytokines and Growth Factors*. New York: Marcel Dekker.
Sporn MB and Roberts AB (1990) *Peptide Growth Factors and their Receptors*, Vols 1 and 2. Berlin: Springer-Verlag.
Thompson A (ed.) (1992) *The Cytokine Handbook*. London: Academic Press.
Walport MJ and Duff GW (1992) Cells and mediators. In: Maddison PJ, Isenberg DA, Woo P and Glass DN (eds) *Oxford Textbook of Rheumatology*. Oxford: Oxford University Press.

8 Skin Lipids

PETER CRITCHLEY

The purpose of this chapter is to focus the attention of the reader on the structure of lipids and how it relates to their function. Skin lipids will be discussed within the framework of structural interactions with a major emphasis on the epidermal barrier lipids, their biosynthesis and problems that occur in skin related to defects in barrier function. Brief mention is made of adipose lipids, sebum in relation to acne, and to apocrine secretion and its associations with pheromonal responses.

HISTORY

Even to our early ancestors, as hunters cooking meat over an open fire, lipids must have been a recognisable part of the diet. The crispy outside or end of a piece of meat is frequently rich in adipose tissue. Moreover, the flammability of the fat dripping from those primitive barbecues was almost certainly noted, leading to the development of candles in later years. Skin and mesenchymal fat mixed with wood ash provided primitive soap, because the alkalinity of the wood ash hydrolysed (saponified) the fats. Moreover, the water-repellent property of lipids was used in waterproofing skins and woven rushes for clothing and the roofs of huts.

More sophisticated mixtures of fats and pigments were used to paint pictures on the walls of caves and as early cosmetic preparations to whiten, darken or colour the skin and hair using natural oxides, carbonates and sulphides of metals such as galena, red iron ore and malachite. The slippery nature of fats did not go unnoticed either and this important property was utilised in lubricating the axles of primitive carts. In later years, a final spark that ignited the Indian mutiny was the use of animal fat to grease gun barrels.

We can conclude that early man understood many of the properties of lipids and used them daily. However, it was several thousand years later, between 1813 and 1825, that a Frenchman called Chevreul determined the structure of fats. He established what happens during saponification and described the structure and properties of most of the major saturated fatty acids from butyric acid with four carbon atoms, through to stearic acid with eighteen carbon atoms.

Molecular Aspects of Dermatology. Edited by G.C. Priestley.
© 1993 by John Wiley & Sons Ltd

DEFINITIONS

The word *lipid* tells one very little about the structure or function of the family of molecules it embraces other than to suggest which solvents might be used to dissolve the molecules. In this respect at least, the generic name is more useful than *carbohydrate*, which only says that the molecules are made up of sugar residues. These may be of several different types, repeated in long chains, soluble or insoluble. Like the carbohydrates, lipids are defined largely on the basis of their chemical structures, properties and functions. The two major classes of lipids are as follows:

(a) *Simple esters* formed through condensation of carboxylic acids and alcohols, which include waxes, animal fats, plant and fish oils; these are almost exclusively composed of carbon, hydrogen and a relatively small percentage of oxygen. The major influence on the properties of these lipids comes from the number of carbon atoms and from the structure of the hydrocarbon tails, i.e. whether they are saturated or unsaturated, branched or straight, short or long.

(b) *More complex esters and amides* include other elements such as nitrogen, phosphorus and sulphur, as well as other classes of molecule such as amino acids, carbohydrates or sterols as part of the molecule. Many of the molecules in this second major class swell on contact with water and their main function is to form interfacial layers or membranes between one environment and another.

The prime function of the class (a) molecules is to act as a food or energy source, although some protective waxes are found in the plant kingdom and fall into this category. The class (b) molecules play many roles but their prime function is to form selective barriers between phases. The permeability of the barrier to passive diffusion can be regulated by the specific composition of the complex lipid mixture that forms the barrier or membrane.

STRUCTURE AND FUNCTION OF LIPIDS

The definition given above is a fairly simple one but can be extended by considering the properties of the lipids and relating these to their functions. A way to illustrate this point is to consider a common fatty acid, stearic acid, which has eighteen carbon atoms arranged as shown in Fig. 8.1. If this molecule is dissolved in a dry organic solvent, such as chloroform, it behaves like a paraffin. However, if we introduce water (which is immiscible with chloroform), the presence of the acid group allows the molecule to interact with water molecules, unlike a paraffin. In fact, the stearic acid groups will pack on the surface of the water with the hydrocarbon tails dissolved in the chloroform and the polar carboxylic acid head groups in the water. So we have a simple

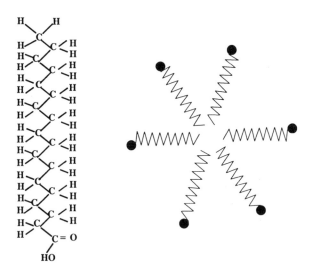

Fig. 8.1. Stearic acid and micelle formation. The full chemical structure of the acid is drawn on the left and a simplified micelle of stearic acid soap in water is shown on the right

interfacial agent trying to form a membrane between chloroform and water. Increasing the polarity of the head groups by making the water solution alkaline will form the soap of stearic acid and this allows the acid to move into water to some extent. As the hydrocarbon tails repel water they are not happy in this solution, so at a relatively low concentration, called the critical micelle concentration (CMC), the molecules associate together, forming micelles or single-layer membranes with all the carboxyl groups pointed outwards into the water and all the hydrocarbon tails pointing inwards protected within the micelle (Fig. 8.1). Many of the lipids in group (b) have more complex structures, such as phospholipids, and are better suited to self-associate into micelles and double-layered membrane-like structures called liposomes (Fig. 8.2).

When a lipid such as stearic acid is mixed with water under neutral or slightly acidic conditions (when it cannot form a soap), it is insoluble and sits at the interfaces of the liquid with the air and also between the liquid and the vessel walls. This is because the properties of unionised stearic acid are totally dominated by the hydrocarbon chain which has no affinity for the water. Stearic acid is a waxy solid, but the properties change slightly to give a liquid at body temperature when pairs of hydrogen atoms are removed from the hydrocarbon tail to produce oleic acid (eighteen carbons with one unsaturation between carbons 9 and 10). Removal of further pairs of hydrogen atoms produces linoleic acid with two unsaturations (at C9 and C12) and lineolic acid with three unsaturations (C9, C12 and C15) which are liquid at room temperature.

The reason for this dramatic change in properties with such a small change in

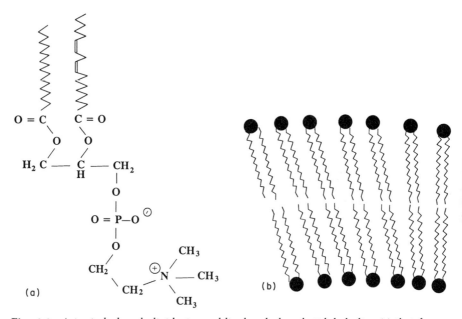

Fig. 8.2. A typical phospholipid, stearoyl linoleoyl phosphatidyl choline (a) that forms flexible or planar bilayers (b) depending on the neutralisation of the head group charge and the fluidity of the hydrocarbon tails

molecular weight is that the hydrocarbon tails in the fully saturated stearic acid pack closely together, whereas the presence of unsaturated bonds interrupts the packing. Closely packed molecules have a degree of crystallinity, forming waxy solids or liquid crystals, whereas chains with interruptions in the sequence, such as double bonds or side branches from the main chain (e.g. isostearic acid), cannot pack closely together and are liquids.

All of the principles described for stearic acid as a representative lipid molecule apply to more complex structures. The presence of two long chains attached to a significant polar head group, e.g. a phospholipid, allows the molecule to form much more stable packed layers, particularly in the presence of other molecules such as cholesterol – a component of many biological membranes. In excess water the typical bilayer structure is assumed, with the polar head groups associating with the water and the tails hidden within the bilayer. When there is very little water the reverse is true; the head groups point inwards to protect the water from the hydrocarbon environment.

The mixture of complex lipid components that are found in the membranes of different living organisms can be understood if one relates some of the membrane functions to the temperature and salinity of the environment. Species growing in Antarctica have many more branched and unsaturated lipid components than those found close to the equator. The presence of high salinity has two main effects: firstly it increases the interaction with water particularly for molecules with carboxyl groups; and secondly it shields the repulsion forces between head groups of more highly charged molecules like phospholipids and allows them to pack more tightly. This would be a disadvantage to a cell, where the surface area of the membrane is optimised for survival. In fact, organisms living in highly saline or high-temperature conditions have developed complex cross-linked, and therefore more rigid, pairs of lipids that have ether-linked branched alkyl chains replacing the more hydrolysable ester linkages (Fig. 8.3). The presence of the branched chains changes the packing of any membrane formed because chains of this type require a larger spatial volume. The presence of a large glycolipid head group with three sugars on it more than compensates for the thicker cross-section of the branched hydrocarbon tails, and mixing three molecules of phospholipid to one of glycolipid adjusts the curvature of the bilayer structure to form a suitable membrane (Kates, 1984).

It is clear from the descriptions above that a complete strategy has evolved for membranes and waxy coats that enables the structures created to function in the widely different environments in which organisms grow. Moreover, membrane compositions do change to allow more or less fluidity depending on the environment of the cells. Thus, more branched and unsaturated fatty acids are found in phospholipids extracted from cells growing at low temperatures because these hydrocarbon tails make the lipids pack less closely and so the membrane is more fluid. In contrast, highly saturated, long straight chains with more than sixteen carbon atoms provide a more waxy and less fluid membrane to operate at slightly higher temperatures. At extremes of salinity and temperature, ether links (which are more stable) replace ester links and some cross-linking of phospholipids, glycolipids and sulpholipids occurs to provide larger and more rigid (less fluid) blocks of membrane components (Kates, 1984).

The concept that changes of structure produce changes in the packing of

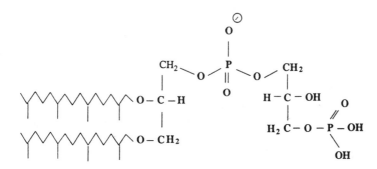

Fig. 8.3. Diphytanyl phosphatidyl glycerophosphate, a membrane component in halophilic organisms. The ether-linked phytanyl tails have a thicker cross-section than normal fatty acid chains because of the methyl side branches. While the two phosphate groups compensate partially for the wider tails, a combination of glycolipid with three sugar groups and phospholipid provides a compact membrane structure resistant to high salt concentration

lipids is critical to understanding why the skin changes from phospholipids to cerebrosides and then to ceramides as one moves from within the body to the outside interface with the environment.

LIPID STRUCTURES AND SECRETIONS IN THE SKIN

So far skin has only been mentioned briefly. If one applies the thinking developed in the section on structure and function of lipids to the main layers of the skin, then a simple table results (Table 8.1).

DERMIS

Dermal connective tissue has few cells compared with epidermis and the main lipids are concentrated in specific glands (which are extensions of the living epidermis and will be discussed later) and in adipose tissue. The adipose, fatty layers are composed mainly of triglycerides that represent a potential energy store when fasting and provide some insulation against cold to maintain the deep body temperature and hence the optimum enzymic functions of the body.

Table 8.1. The types of lipids in different layers of skin and their function

Skin layer	Type of lipid	Function
Adipose tissue	Triglyceride	Food storage and thermal insulation
Dermis		
Basal layer	Phospholipids, cholesterol, small amount of triglyceride	Selective permeability membranes
Spinous layer	Membrane lipids plus lamellar bodies with cerebrosides, cholesterol, fatty acid, triglyceride	Synthesis and organisation of lamellar lipids within cells
Granular layer		
Inner horny layer	Cerebrosides and ceramides, cholesterol, fatty acid, sterol and wax esters	Final enzymic modification of waterproof barrier
Outer horny layer	Lamellar lipids (no cerebrosides)	Barrier
In specific body sites only	Sebum lipids (triglycerides, squalene); apocrine steroids	Smell recognition?
	Extraneous lipids: cosmetics; pollutants	None, but these lipids dissolve in sebum and skin lipid

The exact composition of fatty acids present reflects the diet and the environmental conditions. The composition of lipids in many organisms, including mammals (e.g. pig back-fat), changes depending on the environmental temperature at the time the lipids were stored. Adipose tissue can act as a reservoir of materials that have entered the body and are very soluble in fat. This is particularly true of materials like steroids that are administered topically to the skin.

EPIDERMIS AND SKIN GLANDS

The next major layer of the skin is the epidermis. The lipids in the membranes of the keratinocytes and other cells of the epidermis are typical membrane phospholipids and cholesterol. Some triglycerides are present as oil droplets within the cells and these may represent a potential source of energy to fuel the very active differentiation programme that keratinocytes undergo once they leave the basal layer.

Lipid-soluble materials added to the skin will partition into the membranes and, at non-physiological concentrations, can cause some disturbance to the normal cell membrane function. However, the ability of epidermal tissue to maintain its functions of growth and differentiation has shown that healthy skin can overcome most insults very rapidly. The several glands in the skin can be regarded as extensions of the epithelium as they are almost completely surrounded by a continuous sheath of epithelial cells. The three main glands are the eccrine glands, that function as thermoregulators, secreting mainly water and salts, the sebaceous glands producing lipids, and the apocrine glands producing protein and a variety of steroids. The last two glands are associated with hair follicles, and the distribution and activity of the glands is very different in different parts of the body. Further discussion of eccrine glands is not relevant in this chapter and apocrine glands will be described only briefly.

APOCRINE GLANDS AND BODY ODOURS

Apocrine glands produce a holocrine secretion. That is to say that the cells of the gland continue to divide, grow and accumulate the secretion until they burst, disgorging their contents into the lumen of the gland that connects with the hair follicle. These glands are restricted to specific areas of the body: the axilla, the areolar region of the female breast and the pubic area. Very low volumes of viscous, often slightly yellow secretion are produced, particularly after stimulation of the body to produce adrenal hormones. This can be simulated by intradermal injection of adrenalin.

The composition of the apocrine secretion has not been fully characterised but most of the viscosity is due to a high content of protein. There is very little nucleic acid, so some selective metabolism must occur to recycle valuable nucleotides before rupture of the cell. Much of the mystery of the glands and their secretions revolves around the anatomical location and the widely different mixtures of steroids that are present in the secretion (Critchley, 1993). Many of the steroids are volatile molecules with a musky or peppery odour that is a characteristic high note of underarm odour. At least two of the volatile androstene steroids are known to occur in boar taint, a pheromonal secretion from male pigs that makes the female ready for mounting at the time of insemination. There is no smell from sterile apocrine secretion collected from the human axilla, because the volatile steroids are present as sulphates that must be hydrolysed by enzymes (produced by bacteria on the skin surface) to release the free steroids.

Other molecules, particularly short-chain fatty acids, contribute to all body odours and in many animals it is the particular mixture of different fatty acids present that provides the territorial markers and pack recognition signals. While there is some evidence that babies recognise their mothers by the smell of the nipple (an area of skin with apocrine glands), the evidence suggesting that apocrine glands produce pheromones that are sexual attractants is poor. The steroids are produced to a greater or lesser extent in both men and women, again suggesting the role is not to attract one of the opposite sex. However, women seem more sensitive in detecting the pure compounds and there is a lower frequency of anosmia among women. The apparent anosmic response is not a failure to detect the steroid molecules, because people wired up to a lie detector show an excitation conductivity increase when presented with filter paper strips anointed with the steroids, even when they claim that the particular strip was a blank or control. If the steroids were sex attractants why should they cause this 'excitation' in males who claim not to smell them? It is more likely that these compounds are part of an aggression-signalling response or perhaps a recognition marker for *Homo sapiens*. More work is necessary to sort out these various possibilities.

SEBACEOUS GLANDS AND ACNE

Human sebaceous glands are concentrated mainly on the face, the scalp and the upper torso, and are absent from the palms and the soles of the feet. They produce a holocrine secretion that is mainly neutral lipids (the protein, DNA and phospholipid having been recycled within the gland). The composition of sebum is different for different groups of mammals but is very similar in closely related species.

The gland size and activity are under androgenic hormone control, and in prepubertal human skin the glands are small and most of the sebocytes contain relatively little lipid. In mature glands, the cells increase their volume up to 150-fold with lipid. In young children the composition of sebum is different, containing a much higher proportion of cholesterol (C) and cholesterol esters (CE) compared with wax esters (WE). As the glands are stimulated by androgens (particularly dehydrotesterone) and they mature, the composition changes to 40–57% triglyceride, 25% wax esters, up to 16% free fatty acid, 12% squalene and only 4–5% free sterol plus sterol esters. Free fatty acids are not disgorged by the gland and are produced later by the action of bacterial lipases in the hair canal. The bacterial action is certainly well documented and the free fatty acids were thought to penetrate into, and irritate, the pilosebaceous follicle causing acne (see later in this section).

While the biosynthetic pathways that form the relevant blocks of lipids are relatively standard, the specific profile of sebum lipids is quite different from that of the circulating lipids carried on albumin or of the cell membrane lipids of sebocytes in the gland. Therefore, it is fairly safe to conclude that most of the structures are synthesised locally. In man $\Delta6$-unsaturated palmitic and isopalmitic acids account for almost 70% of the fatty acids, whereas elsewhere in the body the main unsaturated fatty acids are oleic and linoleic acid, which are of $\Delta9$ and $\Delta12$ series of unsaturated acids derived from stearic acid.

The fact that the rate of sebum production (on the scalp about 100 µg of sebum per square centimetre per hour) varies from summer to winter may be explained by seasonal hormonal variations or it may be an artefact of the sampling and analytical method. Sebum flow is influenced to some extent by temperature and the amount of perspiration produced. Therefore, in winter months the flow is slower because of the greater viscosity. After defatting by washing or solvent extraction the surface film is replaced rapidly. However, measurements on the rate of synthesis suggest 8–10 days for [^{14}C]acetate to be incorporated into lipid and appear on the surface of the skin. A possible explanation of the slow replacement is that the surface of the horny layer is hydrophobic and it is crossed by many small crevices. Therefore, lipid from the follicular canal will spread rapidly across the surface because of a favourable interaction with it, particularly along the small crevices. In contrast, water droplets often sit as tight spheres not wetting the surface of skin when soap is not present to form an interface.

Fasting depresses the triglyceride and wax ester content of sebum by 50%, whereas squalene biosynthesis is unchanged and therefore becomes proportionately higher (twice as much). Changes in the composition of sebum have led to the suggestion that the lipid comes from two sources: (a) local synthesis in the gland, which is variable; and (b) a contribution from the circulation and epidermal synthesis that is fairly constant. The lower content of stearic and oleic acis at high rates of sebum secretion could be explained in this way.

The function of sebum was probably associated with more hairy species and may have been a natural conditioning agent for hair. The idea that sebum helps to waterproof the skin is almost certainly incorrect as sebum production is very low in young children and sebum is not a significant barrier to water loss in damaged skin. Indeed the chemical composition is quite different in different animals, and sebum does not contain the right sorts of lipids to form stable barriers or membranes, e.g. phospholipids or sphingolipids. Some components of sebum may be precursors of species-specific odours. It is known that bacterial degradation of lipids in specific anal glands of a number of carnivores produces mixtures of fatty acids that are recognised as markers of dominance and of territory.

ACNE

Acne is the most common disease of the pilosebaceous unit and its appearance is associated with particularly greasy skin in adolescence. However, the high output of sebum is not the sole cause because greasy skin can occur without any sign of acne and indeed is often found in patients whose acne has regressed.

The term acne includes a number of clinically distinct conditions, some of which can progress from one into another. While the common blackheads and whiteheads (open and closed comedones) are not a major problem for most people, papules, which are inflamed lesions that can spread laterally within the skin and may last up to 6 weeks, are very unsightly and cause considerable discomfort and embarrassment. The progression of active papules into nodules can result in scarring of the skin (Cunliffe, 1990).

In spite of the many papers and books written on the subject of acne the mechanisms involved in the pathological changes are still unclear. Acne is certainly androgen mediated and usually appears at puberty. Two major sets of factors are required: (a) high sebum secretion rate; and (b) hypercornification of the ductal epithelium. It is claimed that acne is caused by an interaction between the large amount of sebum, the bacteria that live in the duct and the large number of improperly shed corneocytes that block the duct. Such a mixture is a good recipe for producing potential inflammatory agents, enzymes and antigens and it would be surprising if there was no reaction from the body. However, the initial stimuli that cause hyperproliferation and cornification to occlude the duct have eluded researchers for years.

Topical anti-androgens act directly on sebocytes to reduce both the synthesis of lipid over a period of 3 weeks and the size of the gland over a longer time (2–3 months). In contrast, oestradiol suppresses lipid secretion but has no effect on the mitotic rate of the cells in the gland. The success of anti-androgens, oestrogens and 13-cis-retinoic acid in reducing sebum secretion and improving some forms of acne can be explained if one considers that the linoleic acid in sebum comes from the diet. At high rates of sebum secretion the local production of unsaturated palmitic and isopalmitic acids predominates and therefore the proportion of epidermal and circulatory lipids that contain dietary linoleic acid falls. It was claimed (Downing et al., 1986) that such an adverse change in the proportion of essential fatty acid could produce a local deficiency in the solution that bathes the follicular epithelium. The epithelium would respond with a hyperkeratosis typical of essential fatty acid-deficient skin. Moreover, reduction in the secretion rate with anti-androgens or 13-cis-retinoic acid would restore the level of linoleate and the follicular keratinization would return to normal. This complex of interacting pathways requires much more detailed probing to substantiate the hypothesis.

THE HORNY LAYER AND BARRIER LIPIDS

BARRIER FORMATION

One of the most fascinating features of skin lipids is the very sharp transformation that occurs in the one or two cell layers called the granular layer, i.e. the transition zone between the keratinocytes of the living epidermis and the corneocytes of the horny layer. It is the very active cellular metamorphosis that occurs in and around the granular layer that gives rise to the lipid barrier of the skin. Without this highly impermeable barrier we could not control water loss sufficiently to survive as terrestrial animals. Moreover, contact with many chemicals would cause major responses in our bodies ranging from inflammation to cell death. These are avoided because the barrier controls or prevents

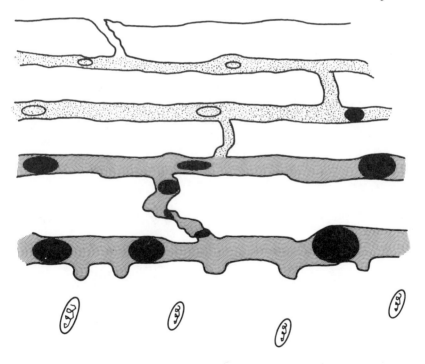

Fig. 8.4. The formation of the stratum corneum as a bricks (corneocytes) and mortar (lamellar lipid) model. The darker shading represents multilamellar lipid between the corneocytes with a greater frequency of intact desmosomes, represented as black oval bodies. Lamellar bodies are represented as oval-shaped bodies with a folded lipid lamellar content. The very irregular membrane on the top of the granular cell represents fusion of lamellar body membranes

penetration of potentially damaging molecules into the vital tissues (Scheup-lein, 1978).

The structure of the skin changes from a close-packed aggregate of more or less cubical cells with conventional phospholipid membranes, communicating with each other freely and with many desmosomes on the cell surfaces binding cells together, to a bricks and mortar structure where the major lipids are between the cells forming the mortar (Fig. 8.4). In fact, desmosomes are still present in the horny layer but fewer of them are detectable in the cells closest to the surface. Moreover, the nuclei and mitochondria that one expects to see within highly metabolically active cells have largely disappeared. The cells become elongated, flattened and filled with folded sheets of keratin, which gives each cell a significant rigidity. The main changes in lipid composition are the replacement of phospholipids by ceramides, an increase in free sterol and a large increase in free fatty acid at the expense of triglyceride and phospholipid (Table 8.1). This transformation of the lipid provides the outer layers of the skin with a much more stable, waxy and impermeable lipid barrier.

The barrier is not just a single band of lipid like a conventional membrane but ramifies right through the horny layer. The components of the barrier are mainly composed of carbon–carbon bonds and are therefore much more stable to enzymes, ultraviolet light, oxidation and temperature differences than conventional esters and phospholipids.

The lamellar phase-forming lipids of the horny layer are not phospholipids but are long-chain (C22 to C30) ceramides with small head groups of two or three hydroxyl groups and an amide link. Indeed ceramide I, the least polar of

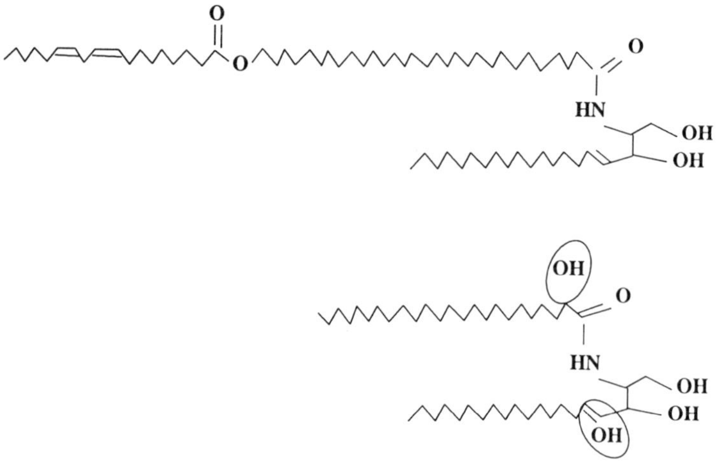

Fig. 8.5. Ceramide I, an acylated ω-hydroxy ceramide, is shown on the top and a more typical ceramide structure is shown below. The hydroxyl groups and double bond in the rings are variations of the structures found in human skin

the six classes of the ceramides found in skin, is unique to epidermal tissue (Fig. 8.5). It has a longer than average ω-hydroxy acid forming the normal amide bond with sphingosine or sphingenine. The ω-OH position is esterified with fatty acids, and in human skin linoleic acid makes up 50% of the ω-hydroxy ester. The asymmetry of the chains produces some different properties from those of the other ceramides. Recent work in the author's laboratory has suggested that the molecule may play a crucial role in plasticising the horny layer to allow stretching and bending by fluidising the barrier lipids (Rawlings *et al.*, 1993). In the skin of marine mammals and in non-keratinising epithelium the fatty acid chain lengths are shorter and glycosyl units are not removed from the sphingosine. More polar lipids than occur in human horny layer are found mixed into the membrane structure to provide a working membrane, but one which permits a relatively high water flux.

The cellular processes affecting the lipid transformation are very interesting. One might ask, how does the body assemble a specific, insoluble, waxy lipid phase in the horny layer? The answer is that the cells don't assemble the lipid mixture in the horny layer. What actually happens is that lamellar bodies develop within the spinous cells and these continue to fill with precursor lipids as they pass into the granular layer. At this stage the lipid bodies occupy up to 25% of the cytosol and contain clearly recognisable lamellae of lipid showing electron-dense and electron-lucent bands with characteristic spacing for bilayers and double bilayers. X-ray crystallographic evidence has confirmed the existence of these structures.

It was thought that the lamellae were separate discs of lipid which fused together after secretion from the cells of the granular layer. However, recent evidence has shown that the lamellae are connected together as a folded concertina and that they unfold on secretion (Elias and Menon, 1991). Moreover, the lipid composition within the lamellar body and at the time of secretion is more mobile than that found nearer to the surface of the horny layer. The limiting membrane that contained the lamellar bodies is spliced into the envelope of the granular cell, increasing the surface area/volume ratio significantly. This may explain why the horny layer can absorb up to four times its own weight of water without the cells bursting. The corneocytes contain a variety of humectants and natural sunscreening agents that are synthesised from proteins, many of which are specially built up during the maturation and differentiation of keratinocytes. It is these molecules in particular that absorb the water. The cell envelope of the corneocytes is believed to be lipoprotein and to be cross-linked to ceramide molecules that form the first layer of the multilamellar lipid present in the intercellular spaces. Extraction of the horny layer with a good solvent for lipids, such as chloroform, removes much of the more loosely associated intercellular lipid layers, and only a thin band of residual lipid, possibly that bound to the cell surface, remains (Fig. 8.6).

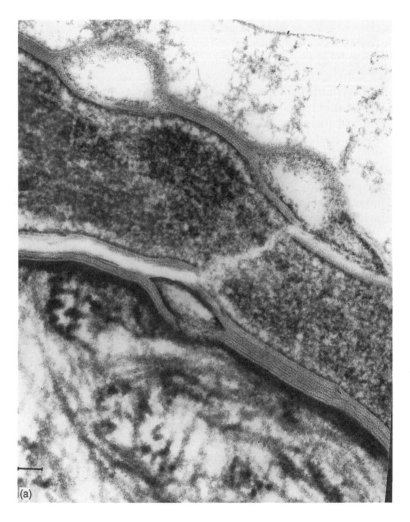

Fig. 8.6. Electron micrograph of ruthenium tetroxide fixed and stained horny layer showing the multilamellar lipid layers between individual corneocytes (a) and the removal of much of the lipid structure by extraction with solvent (b). The electron microscopy was done by Mr J. Hope. The bar is 0.05 μm

A number of enzymes are released at the same time as the lipids, and further modify the structure of some of them to produce a mixture with far less affinity for water. The four most notable changes are:

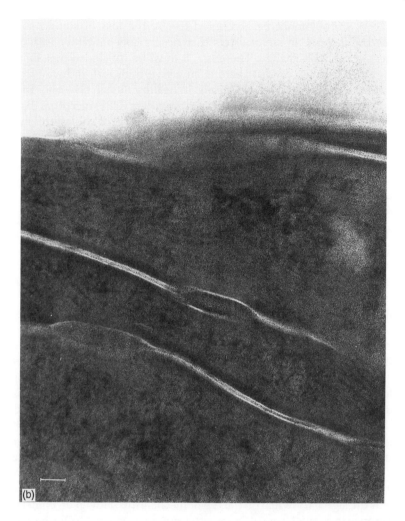

(a) The conversion of glucosyl ceramides (cerebrosides) into ceramides by a specific glucosidase, thereby reducing the polarity or size of the head group significantly.
(b) The more than doubling of the percentage of free fatty acids at the expense of triglycerides and phospholipids, which are degraded by lipases and phospholipases.
(c) The almost doubling of the proportion of free sterol.
(d) The halving of the proportion of cholesterol sulphate, resulting from the action of a steroid sulphatase. It is interesting that neither the steroid sulphate nor the sulphatase enzyme concentrates within lamellar bodies but both are in the intercellular lipid close to corneocyte envelopes.

The excess sterol cannot be accounted for by the loss of steroid sulphate, because the increase in sterol esters that occurs concomitantly would more than account for this change. Therefore, it must be concluded that significant local synthesis occurs or that there is an active transport pathway from the vasculature through the vital epidermis. In healthy human skin only the basal layers of the epidermis have low-density lipoprotein (LDL) receptors that carry cholesterol to cell membranes, and the circulating level of cholesterol in blood has no effect on *de novo* cholesterol synthesis, suggesting that transport through the epidermis is low.

REGULATION OF BIOSYNTHETIC RATES AND RESPONSE TO DAMAGE

The rate of cholesterol synthesis is controlled by modulation of the rate-limiting enzyme 3-hydroxy-3-methylglutaryl coenzyme A (HMG-CoA) reductase in keratinocytes. In turn, this enzyme responds to both LDL receptor binding in the basal cells and particularly to increases in water flux through an impaired barrier, caused by solvent or essential nutrient imbalances, e.g. essential fatty acid deficiency. The switching on and off of increased cholesterol synthesis is rapid and the return to normal balance occurs within 24 hours unless the skin has suffered serious damage, e.g. severe exposure to cold, dry conditions or excessive sunburn. The skin may need several days to recover from more serious disruptions and topical application of creams helps by providing a barrier while the skin repairs itself by mitosis and differentiation.

Rates of fatty acid release are very similar to the time–response curves produced for cholesterol in the case of acute barrier disruption, and chronic changes caused by essential fatty acid deficiency. However, sphingolipid production is not triggered immediately after solvent damage but starts several hours later. Occlusion of the skin prevents all of these repair processes and it is tempting to think that the increased flux of water resulting from a defective barrier is the signal to switch on the repair mechanisms. However, immersion of hairless mice in a variety of solutions, after previous damage to the barrier with acetone, did not prevent repair. Only solutions of calcium or potassium salts were able to inhibit repair, suggesting that specific signalling channels in the membranes of keratinocytes may be a major site of control (Feingold, 1991).

The time–response curves for barrier repair and the rate-limiting enzymes involved in the biosynthetic pathways have been elegantly demonstrated by the use of specific inhibitors of these enzymes (Feingold, 1991). Thus, topical lovastatin inhibits HMG-CoA reductase (hence cholesterol synthesis) for several hours, causing barrier disruption but allowing other lipids to accumulate. Simultaneous administration of topical cholesterol repairs the barrier. If lovastatin treatment is continued to establish a chronic situation, then the lamellar bodies are abnormal and some fail to secrete the lipid lamellae, possibly producing an uneven barrier distribution.

Similarly, β-chloroalanine has been used to inhibit serine palmitoyl transferase, the rate-limiting enzyme in the biosynthesis of ceramides. Again, barrier function is impaired but only after 12–24 hours. The addition of ceramide topically overcomes the β-chloroalanine blockade.

Disruption of the barrier not only triggers a rapid biosynthetic repair cascade, but DNA synthesis and subsequent mitosis can also be demonstrated. The extent of the DNA synthesis correlates with the degree of barrier disruption and again occlusion prevents the activation of the synthetic process, in this case DNA synthesis. Such observations could be highly relevant to the dressing of burns and other skin damage and may also explain why submerged cultures of skin do not differentiate properly, particularly when the probes used for differentiation are biochemical and immunological markers rather than histological ones.

CONDITIONS OF THE SKIN THAT MAY BE RELATED TO BARRIER FUNCTION

It is difficult and scientifically unwise to relate an accumulation of changes diagnosed clinically as a disease to a single biochemical or structural molecular change, unless one can reproduce the clinical symptoms by effecting the single change.

Abnormalities of the skin, not related to glands or pilosebaceous ducts, fall into two broad groups:

(a) Those involving excessive division of keratinocytes, frequently coupled with incomplete differentiation so that the living epidermis is thickened as well as the horny layer.
(b) A specific thickening of the horny layer, with no obvious change in epidermal turnover or rate of progression of keratinocytes into the granular layer. In this latter group the major abnormality is a low rate of desquamation, frequently coupled with the loss of large scales of many cells rather than individual corneocytes.

As was mentioned much earlier in this chapter, a major disturbance of the barrier function will expose the body to numerous insults and stimuli from the environment, to which the body will then respond appropriately. Therefore, once the barrier function is compromised many of the symptoms observed are the result of chemicals and antigens to which the body was exposed. This is one reason why it is difficult to relate disease symptoms of skin to a specific single cause.

A further difficulty is the fact that genetic deficiencies are often not specific to skin, and similar molecules to those found in the skin occur in other areas of the body. Thus, the membranes of nerve cells and brain are compiled from a range of phospholipids, galactosyl ceramides and cholesterol. Any widespread genetic defect in the synthesis of any of these lipids could cause major metabolic imbalances in several areas of the body that could have indirect as well as direct effects on the skin. A change in hormonal or neuropeptide balance resulting from changed sensitivities of the membranes of nervous tissue might be expected to produce symptoms in remote tissues under constant challenge like the skin and the gastrointestinal system. For the same reasons, a number of temporary disturbances in metabolism caused by stress, infection, allergy or imbalanced nutrition can result in 'transient' symptoms clinically diagnosed in the skin.

Table 8.2. The relationship between changes in skin structure and lipid metabolism

Skin problem	Changes in lipid
Acute damage causing barrier breakdown, e.g. solvent or detergent exposure. Dry skin	Loss of some ceramide, cholesterol, fatty acid, wax and sterol esters from barrier. Replacement by synthesis initially of cholesterol and fatty acid
Chronic damage caused by essential fatty acid deficiency or hypocholesterolaemic drug. Thickened, dry, scaly corneum	Abnormal lamellar bodies and lamellae. Relative increase in fatty acid synthesis
Genetic defects	
(a) Recessive X-linked ichthyosis	Defect in steroid sulphatase production. Cholesterol sulphate accumulates and poor desquamation results
(b) Refsum disease. Neurological symptoms and ichthyosis	Defect in phytanic acid oxidase production. Branched chain acids spoil packing in membrane lipids
(c) Harlequin ichthyosis	Defect in lamellar bodies which produce and secrete lipid that is too polar. Liposomes formed instead of lamellar plates
(d) Sjögren–Larsson syndrome. Nerves, brain and skin membranes	Fatty alcohol oxidoreductase deficiency leads to abnormal membranes. Ether lipids made from fatty alcohols are stable to lipases
(e) CHILD syndrome, Conradi–Hünermann type and rhizomelic type chondrodysplasia punctata	Defect in peroxisome lipid metabolism, particularly phytanic acid oxidation and plasmologen synthesis
(f) Neutral lipid storage disease. Generalised triglyceride accumulation in many organs and skin ichthyosis	Defect most likely in lipase that facilitates phospholipid synthesis from triglyceride

It is worth summarising the known disturbances to lipid metabolism within the skin so that the reader can relate the structure and function of the lipids to real dermatological problems (Table 8.2).

ACUTE DAMAGE

The effects of acute damage caused by solvents, harsh detergents or sunlight directly to the skin barrier and to the living epidermal cells responsible for repairing or replacing the barrier have been described under the section on barrier formation.

CHRONIC DAMAGE

Hypocholesterolaemic agents such as lovastatin (see earlier) are known to induce poor barrier function and scaling of the skin surface if used for a significant time. These drugs block cholesterol synthesis within the epidermis, and cholesterol is a vital part of the membrane lipid.

A further chronic problem in the past was directly associated with essential fatty acid deficiency in patients undergoing prolonged lipid-free parenteral nutrition. The human body cannot make its own linoleic acid, despite the fact that this acid is accumulated specifically in the barrier lipids, particularly in the ω-hydroxy acid esters. Moreover, the acid is the normal precursor for the synthesis of arachidonic acid, which when liberated from phospholipids in membranes is converted into the two families of eicosanoids. Arachidonic acid and cyclooxygenases produce prostaglandins, whereas lipoxygenases act on arachidonic acid to produce hydroxy acids. When linoleic acid is deficient in the diet, oleic acid is incoporated into lipids like ceramide I as a replacement. The lamellar bodies of the skin are incomplete or only partially filled, water flux is high, the skin is more permeable to water-soluble molecules and scaling dermatitis results. It is known that eicosanoids are produced by keratinocytes and it is thought that at least one factor regulating cell turnover may be the concentration of these pharmacologically active molecules. In linoleic acid-deficient skin, hyperproliferation occurs and eicosanoid production will be very low or absent. Topical application of prostaglandin E2 or arachidonic acid to essential fatty acid-deficient skin inhibits the dermatitis but has no effect on barrier function. In contrast, linoleic acid applied topically or systemically improves the barrier function. Indeed this occurs even when the eicosanoid pathways are deliberately blocked by the use of cyclooxygenase and lipoxygenase inhibitors. Barrier function can be improved by topical application of two related unsaturated acids to linoleic acid, i.e. those having unsaturations at carbons 5 and 8 or 6 and 9. These acids are not metabolised to eicosanoids but will form barrier esters.

A form of atopic eczema responds well to a systemic mixture of evening primrose oil that contains linoleic acid and γ-linoleic acid and safflower oil that is rich in linoleic acid. It is thought that inositol phosphates are liberated from inositol phospholipids and these second messengers help to normalise hyperproliferation caused by the deficiency in essential fatty acids.

GENETIC DISORDERS

Several genetic disorders can be related to defects in lipid metabolism (Table 8.2). In a number of these examples the detailed mechanism is unknown, whereas in others it is fairly clear.

Recessive X-linked ichthyosis

The skin appears to be normal at birth in this condition but scaling starts after a few weeks. There is no major increase in epidermal turnover and the symptoms point to a defect in the desquamation process. Biochemically there is a large increase (up to fivefold) in the proportion of cholesterol sulphate in the skin, particularly in the granular layer, but a significant amount of this sterol sulphate is retained in the horny layer. The genetic defect has been shown to be a lesion in the sterol sulphatase gene so that minimal levels of the enzyme are produced in the skin. The overall proportion of sterol sulphate, sterol esters and free sterol to other lipids does not change, but the free sterol content is low. The barrier function is slightly less efficient but there is no dramatic change.

While cholesterol sulphate diffuses through skin fairly freely and can inhibit HMG-CoA reductase at physiological concentrations, this does not seem to be the major mechanism because the cholesterol concentration is only reduced by a factor of two and the barrier function, which is known to be highly sensitive to cholesterol depletion (see lovastatin inhibition above), is only slightly impaired. Therefore, the delayed desquamation is probably better explained by an alternative mechanism. Cholesterol sulphate has been shown to be a very powerful inhibitor of a serine protease in the sperm membrane. Sulphatase in the female reproductive tract hydrolyses the sulphate, removing the blockade on the protease, which can in turn prepare the membrane for fusion. It is possible that a parallel mechanism operates in horny layer desquamation (Williams, 1991). Circumstantial evidence supporting this hypothesis is the fact that 5–20% of the total lipid in the hoof of ungulates is cholesterol sulphate and that this tissue is very difficult to disrupt because the cells stick together very well. A further piece of evidence is that cholesterol sulphate applied topically to animal skin causes scaling, strongly suggesting a local effect upon desquamation.

Refsum disease

This is a rare autosomal recessive disorder that affects nerve tissue as well as causing ichthyotic skin. The disease develops progressively and can be correlated with the phytol (plant chlorophyll component) intake. Indeed, phytanic acid oxidase has been shown to be deficient in patients suffering from this condition and significant accumulations of phytanic acid are found in the lipid fractions, e.g. up to 45% in phospholipids and 35% in sterol esters.

The significant increase in the cross-sectional diameter of the phytanyl chains (because of the methyl side branches, see Fig. 8.3) over linear hydrocarbons will disrupt membrane packing, unless some large polar head group (three or four sugar residues) are incorporated into a proportion of the lamellar lipids to balance the spatial demands of the bulky tails. There are histological reports that large lipid vacuoles are present in epidermal cells, probably because their membranes are faulty. The response of the skin is likely to be a significant thickening to compensate for poor barrier qualities and this is indeed what happens. However, changes occur to membranes around and within many cells throughout the body and therefore this is a case where very careful interpretation and further investigation are necessary before one can draw conclusions.

Harlequin ichthyosis

This autosomal recessive disorder is obvious from birth and frequently fatal. The horny layer looks like the large plate-like scales of a fish or lizard. Eating and respiratory movements are difficult. The evidence points to a defect in the formation of the lamellar bodies in the spinous layer. Lipid vacuoles and unusual membranes with concentric lamellar structures are present in the granular layer and many of the lipid bodies are retained in the horny layer instead of being secreted into the intercellular lipid domains between the corneocytes. The concentric lamellar structures are formed by lamellar lipids with large head groups in an aqueous environment, so one might expect phospholipid (including the more polar phosphatidylinositol) and glycosyl ceramides to be major components of these liposome-like structures. The exact mechanisms have not been identified.

Sjögren–Larsson syndrome

This is another condition involving a number of tissues including nerves, brain and skin. The autosomal recessive syndrome was identified in in-bred groups in the north of Sweden. The main lesion is a deficiency of the fatty alcohol oxidoreductase that should convert fatty alcohol into fatty acid. Restricting the diet to medium-chain-length triglycerides helps to alleviate some of the symptoms, particularly the ichthyosis. At present it is impossible to speculate what the mechanism is or how many different pathways are involved.

CHILD syndrome, Conradi–Hünermann type and rhizomelic type chondrodysplasia punctata

The diseases in this group have one thing in common: they all result from genetic lesions in peroxisomes, the intracellular organelles that process so many of the chemicals passing through a cell. The significance for this chapter is that the oxidation of phytanic acid (mentioned above) and the dihydroxyacetone phosphate acyltransferase that catalyses the first step in plasmalogen synthesis is deficient. In at least some of these disorders the main lesion occurs in fibroblasts in the dermis rather than in the keratinocytes. The biochemistry of the diseases is poorly understood and awaits further research.

Neutral lipid storage disease

The genetic lesion(s) in neutral lipid storage disease (NLSD) result in a widespread accumulation of triglycerides in non-membrane-bound cytoplasmic droplets. Symptoms occur in many organs and include neurosensory deafness, cataracts, fatty liver, clinical myopathy and ichthyosis. While the metabolic defect is unknown, it has been shown that exogenously derived triglycerides accumulate. Homogenised cells possess lipases that degrade all the glycerides, so one has to look to some compartmental problem within the cell. Isolated cell lines, from patients with NLSD, pulsed with [^{14}C]acetate showed an abnormal increase in labelled phosphatidylcholine and ethanolamine (Williams et al., 1991). It was suggested that the genetic problem was a lipase converting newly synthesised glycerides into diacyl glycerol which is rapidly converted to phospholipid.

It is prudent to finish the chapter with a cautionary tale. As the cells move from the epidermis to the horny layer there is a very large shift in lipid composition that is easy to analyse in healthy skin. Further changes occur throughout the horny layer to the skin surface which are much more difficult to analyse and interpret, because the more loosely packed surface layers of the horny layer act as a sponge. They absorb lipid from a variety of sources and this is mixed with the normal corneum lipids forming the barrier. These sources include:

(a) Sebum (in appropriate areas of skin).
(b) Apocrine steroids (in specific areas only).
(c) Deliberately applied creams and lotions.
(d) Components of foam baths, shampoos and other detergents to which the body is exposed.
(e) Lipids of general exogenous origin that partition into the skin lipids by direct contact or from the air.

The author has had experience of both cases (d) and (e). When a large volume of skin washings was collected from armpits to analyse the specific fatty acids and steroids, an apparently new steroid was found. More thorough chemical analysis coupled with mass spectrometry showed that this molecule was not a steroid at all but a foam booster used in the shower gel that the volunteer panellists were using. On another occasion there was great excitement in the laboratory about a completely new lipid found in hair sebum. Once again, however, thorough chemical analysis showed this material to be a plasticiser, used by most of the utility car manufacturers of the time in the seat covers. A statistically significant correlation was obtained between the concentration of the material present and the frequency of riding in relatively new cars.

It is easy to sample the skin surface layers but even easier to be misled by what one thinks one has found there!

REFERENCES

Critchley P (1993) Human pheromones: do they exist? *Journal of the Society of Cosmetic Chemists* (in press).

Cunliffe WJ (1989) *Acne.* Focal Points in Dermatology Series. London: Martin Dunitz.

Downing DT, Stewart ME, Wertz PW and Strauss JS (1986) Essential fatty acids and acne. *Journal of the American Academy of Dermatology* **14**, 215–221.

Elias PM and Menon GK (1991) Structural and lipid biochemical correlates of the epidermal permeability barrier. Ed. Elias PM. *Advances in Lipid Research. Vol. 24, Skin Lipids*, Academic Press, **24**, 1–26.

Feingold KR (1991) The regulation of epidermal lipid synthesis. *Advances in Lipid Research* **24**, 57–82.

Kates M (1984) Adventures in membrane land. *Journal of the American Oil Chemists Society* **61**, 1826–1834.

Rawlings AV, Critchley P, Ackerman C, Parnell A, Rogers J and Oldroyd J (1993) The functional roles of ceramide-one. *Journal of the Society of Cosmetic Chemists* (in press).

Scheuplein R (1978) The skin as a barrier. In: Jarrett A (ed.) *The Physiology and Pathophysiology of the Skin*, Vol. 5, pp. 1669–1692. New York: Academic Press.

Williams ML (1991) Lipids in normal and pathological desquamation. *Advances in Lipid Research* **24**, 211–262.

Williams ML, Coleman RA, Placzek D and Grunfeld C (1991) Neutral lipid storage disease: a possible functional defect in phospholipid linked triacylglycerol metabolism. *Biochimica et Biophysica Acta* **1096**, 162–169.

FURTHER READING

Aloia RC and Boggs JM (1985) *Membrane Fluidity in Biology. Vol. 4, Cellular Aspects.* New York: Academic Press.

Cunliffe WJ (1989) *Acne.* Focal Points in Dermatology Series. London: Martin Dunitz.

Elias PM (1991) *Advances in Lipid Research. Vol. 24, Skin Lipids.* San Diego: Academic Press.

Israelachvili JN (1985) *Intramolecular and Surface Forces with Application to Colloidal and Biological Systems.* San Diego: Academic Press.

Marks R and Christophers E (1981) *The Epidermis in Disease.* Lancaster, UK: MTP Press.

Mead JF, Alfin-Slater RB, Howton DR and Popj'ak G (1986) *Lipids, Chemistry, Biochemistry and Nutrition.* London: Plenum Press.

Solomon AK and Karnovsky M (1978) *Molecular Specialization and Symmetry in Membrane Function.* Cambridge, MA: Harvard University Press.

9 Molecular Genetics of Skin Disease

JONATHAN L. REES

Although the principles of genetics may not have changed much over the last few decades, the growth of recombinant DNA technology has revolutionised both the style and the power of a genetic approach to disease. Much of this growth has been technology driven, in that breakthroughs at a technical level have allowed studies and experiments that were simply inconceivable only a few years earlier. A good example of this has been the invention of the polymerase chain reaction (PCR). The PCR technique, by allowing amplification from a single molecule of DNA to the microgram quantity, has spawned a variety of techniques which were not even imagined only five or six years earlier.

The present chapter is intended not as a catalogue of genetic disorders of the skin – a variety of texts already serve that function. Instead, it attempts to describe the technical changes and novel experimental strategies that now make study of human skin disease easier and more accessible than ever before. The chapter is divided into three sections: firstly, a description of the techniques that underpin the study of the molecular genetics of skin; secondly, an examination of the aims of recombinant DNA work; and thirdly, examples or case studies of the various approaches, successful or otherwise, which are being used to help understand human skin disease.

TECHNIQUES

Chromosomal DNA is the major genetic material of the mammalian cell: mitochondria have their own DNA and, although this has recently been shown to be important in a variety of diseases, it has limited relevance to human skin disease and will not be discussed further. If a small 6 mm punch biopsy of human skin is incubated in a 1.5 ml tube overnight with a potent proteinase such as proteinase K, based on the fact that protein and nucleic acid will differentially partition in an aqueous/phenol mixture, proteins and nucleic acid separate; the resulting sticky, viscous aqueous solution will contain high-molecular-weight DNA and will be largely free of protein. If this aqueous phase is removed and mixed with an equal volume of an alcohol, such as

Molecular Aspects of Dermatology. Edited by G.C. Priestley.
© 1993 by John Wiley & Sons Ltd

isopropanol, a yellowish substance consisting of pure high-molecular-weight DNA will stick to the base of a glass rod placed in this solution. The 50–100 mg or so of DNA isolated can be gently suspended in water and, based on the characteristic absorption spectra of DNA, assayed spectrophotometrically.

Each cell of the body contains 23 pairs of chromosomes, whose DNA molecules, if laid end to end, would total approximately 3×10^{-9} base pairs. The sticky yellow substance around the bottom of the glass rod will therefore consist of DNA molecules totalling 3×10^{-9} bases multiplied by the 10 to 100 million or so cells that have been used to make DNA. The technical revolution has been to develop assays for the functional characteristics of this DNA, which are dependent on its sequence.

The four bases that occur in DNA – two purines and two pyrimidines – bind to each other in a specific manner: guanine with cytosine, and adenine with thiamine, joining the two anti-parallel strands. It is the linear sequence of the bases that is primarily important in determining the information carried by DNA: sequence information from a gene is copied into complementary RNA (messenger RNA) which then in association with ribosomes and transfer RNA allows triplets of DNA bases to determine the primary structure of a particular protein. Even at this stage, it is important to note that the greater part of the DNA stuck to the bottom of the glass rod in the test tube will not consist of protein-coding DNA, but non-coding DNA, or junk DNA, the function of which is still unclear. Nevertheless, any meaningful study of DNA must rely on assays based on the sequence characteristics of the DNA, including of course direct sequencing of individual DNA molecules. Whole volumes are devoted to describing the techniques that allow such analysis of DNA. However, the principles underpinning these techniques are relatively straightforward, and with a minimum of technical information it is intuitively possible to see that much of the power of recombinant DNA technology results from the way in which a relatively small number of techniques are linked together in complex protocols. In any discussion concerning the strategy used by molecular biologists and molecular geneticists it is important to have at least some understanding of these techniques.

Restriction enzymes are enzymes that cut or cleave DNA in a sequence-specific manner. They have been identified, purified and now cloned from a variety of bacteria, and their principal function seems to have been to digest foreign (invading) DNA. (They protect their own DNA from digestion by methylation of some of the bases.) If the DNA at the bottom of the glass rod is gently dissolved in water and incubated with a particular restriction enzyme for a few hours, the large DNA molecules (upwards of 30 000 bases long) will be broken up into smaller pieces in a site- and therefore sequence-dependent manner. There are now hundreds of different restriction enzymes whose sequence requirements differ, and, importantly, the frequency with which these enzymes will cut eukaryotic DNA will depend on the specificity requirements of that particular enzyme. Therefore enzymes such as *EcoR1* will cut whenever they encounter the sequence GAATTC, whereas other enzymes, such as *Not1*, deemed rare cutters, will only cut when they find the sequence GCGGCCGC. Importantly, restriction enzymes often cleave DNA in such a way that it is possible to recreate the site through which the enzyme has cut. This characteristic assumes great importance when particular genes are cloned into *vectors*, allowing large copy numbers to be made of a particular sequence. A DNA molecule, perhaps 1–3 kb long, which has been cut through a particular restriction enzyme site, can be inserted into a circular *plasmid* vector which has also been cut with the same enzyme. When the ends are ligated or stuck together, a new recombinant circular plasmid is created containing the gene of interest. Plasmids are naturally occurring, extra-chromosomal circular DNA found in bacteria, and amongst other things they carry genes coding for antibiotic resistance. In practice, plasmids are a commonly used vector and, by chemically treating the walls of bacteria in such a way that they are made permeable to plasmids, plasmids can be introduced or *transfected* into a variety of bacterial hosts. The bacteria can then be cultured overnight in a suitable medium and the plasmids will replicate with each division of the bacterial cell. Because of the difference in size between plasmid DNA and chromosomal DNA, the plasmid DNA is easily separated, and the gene of interest can now be cut out of the plasmid with the same restriction enzyme that was used to place it in the plasmid. Amongst other things, cloning of the gene in this manner produces large amounts of a particular DNA molecule which is suitable for sequencing or for labelling as a DNA probe.

DNA polymerases are a class of enzyme which, depending on their characteristics, allow copies of nucleic acids to be made. A DNA-dependent DNA polymerase will make complementary copies of each strand of a particular double-stranded DNA molecule. Amongst other things, poly-merases require a primer or short sequence of complementary DNA, usually less than 20 bases long, from which to start the synthesis of the complementary copy. If one of the bases in the buffer medium is radioactive, the polymerase will incorporate this base into the synthesised complementary molecules, and therefore the copies made will be radioactive. This process therefore allows labelled sequence-specific DNA probes to be made.

The DNA which adhered to the bottom of the glass rod and which has been digested with a suitable restriction enzyme can now be size fractionated through an agarose gel. Small amounts of DNA (5–20 µg) are loaded into a small hole (well) at one end of a 20 cm × 20 cm × 1 cm 1% agarose gel. DNA will migrate at a rate inversely proportional to its molecular weight through an electric field applied to the gel. The resulting DNA smear can then be transferred from the agarose on to nylon, by placing a nylon square on top of the gel, together with blotting paper on top of the nylon. Buffer fluid will then move from the gel through the nylon to the blotting paper, transferring the

DNA molecules by capillary action only from the gel to the nylon membrane. One can see intuitively that a gene situated anywhere in the human genome, when cut with a particular restriction enzyme, will migrate through the gel according to its size and the presence or otherwise of the particular restriction enzyme sites, either within the gene or in closely adjacent DNA. This specific migratory pattern will be transferred to the nylon membrane (Southern transfer). If this nylon membrane is now mixed or hybridised with a particular gene probe labelled with radioisotope, as outlined above, then the position of this gene amongst the total smear of DNA can be identified. Because the DNA from different individuals is not absolutely identical, in that variations in sequence will occur between every 1 in 200 to every 1 in 500 bases (polymorphisms), it is possible that individual differences in sequence information may be reflected in different band patterns or position of the bands on the Southern blot (restriction fragment length polymorphisms, RFLPs).

Another use of cloning the DNA molecule of interest into plasmids is to produce large amounts of a particular sequence which could then form the basis for DNA sequencing. Again the principles of DNA sequencing are straightforward, relying on the copying of a particular DNA sequence by a polymerase, only in this case the bases, which again are radioactively labelled, are mixed with a variety of bases that cause the copy of the DNA to terminate prematurely. These aborted transcripts will therefore reveal themselves as shortened DNA molecules (prematurely terminated), and if the results of the reaction are then run on a polyacrylamide gel, a ladder of lines reflecting the primary sequence characteristics of the target DNA will be seen. Although plasmids are widely used as cloning agents, over the last few years another technique, the PCR, has found increasing use in producing large amounts of a particular DNA molecule suitable for sequencing. The principles underlying the PCR are quite simple. A variety of thermostable DNA polymerases, in the presence of sequence-specific primers (i.e. short sequences of DNA complementary to each of the two strands of DNA), will make complementary copies of each strand of the DNA molecules. These complementary copies will re-anneal, but if separated by heating to above 90 °C and then rapidly cooled, will in turn be able to act as templates for more DNA synthesis by the thermostable DNA polymerase. Intuitively, one can see that this amplification will, depending on an adequate supply of reagents, increase the number of target molecules logarithmically. The advantage of this technique is that in theory, and in practice in some hands, only one target molecule is required, although it is usual and desirable to start with more than this, and amplification up to microgram quantities of the desired DNA sequence can be obtained overnight using an automated DNA thermal cycler.

The above techniques form the basis of much of molecular genetics. Although each of them appears very different, at a technical level the sorts of manipulations required are similar and it is the juxtaposition of these techniques into complex protocols that provides much of the power of molecular genetics. It is, however, important to note that scale in these reactions is all important. The crude DNA extracted from the skin sample described earlier needs to be processed in such a way, and into certain size fragments, that sequencing, for instance, is manageable. It is simply impossible to mix all the DNA and sequence 3×10^{-9} base pairs. Usually therefore, for this purpose, the DNA molecules may have to be separated or isolated by cloning into plasmids or other vectors (forming a genomic library where each 'book' represents a single DNA insert inside the vector), so that individual sequences of 500–1000 bases can be subjected to sequencing. Alternatively and increasingly commonly, PCR of individual regions of a few hundred bases will form a basis for DNA sequencing. It is technically demanding to amplify DNA fragments of more than two or three kilobases using the PCR. Therefore a crucial problem lies in marrying conventional genetic mapping techniques and the molecular techniques described above, bridging the gap between centimorgans and bases. For instance, one centimorgan, which represents crossing over occurring in 1% of meioses, may represent one million base pairs. Given that sequence analysis will require DNA fragments of perhaps half a kilobase to a few kilobases in length, one can see that much of the difficulty and therefore technical ingenuity relies on bridging the gap between an area of a chromosome to which a disease has been mapped, and identifying and isolating the particular gene. For these reasons much attention is now focused on particular techniques, such as pulsed field gel electrophoresis, a technique allowing particularly large DNA molecules to be fractionated on agarose gels, and the development of high-density genetic maps based on non-coding sequences, such as microsatellite sequences distributed frequently throughout the genome.

MOLECULAR GENETICS OF SKIN DISEASE: AIMS

It is self-evident that dermatologists and other physicians will wish to treat patients with cutaneous disease more effectively. Therefore at one level the aims of any research into the molecular genetics of skin disease will be to improve current therapy, and if possible prevent cutaneous disease. While acknowledging the undoubted power of much of recombinant DNA technology, but also attempting to take a realistic view of future trends, it is important to think through how improvements in this field will assist in the clinical care of patients. How will the cloning and characterisation and sequencing of the gene that is thought to cause a particular disease assist in patient care? Obviously if the disease is severe, and one can think of the dystrophic forms of epidermolysis bullosa as examples, prenatal diagnosis based on PCR amplification and mutant detection will allow selective termination of pregnancy, if thought appropriate by physician and family. Alternatively, if systems can be invented that will allow for gene therapy, and limited successes have already been reported, direct insertion of recombinant genes into the patient may correct a diseased phenotype.

Nevertheless, in view of the clinical course of most cutaneous diseases, especially with respect to morbidity and mortality, it is clear that these approaches are always going to be peripheral to most clinical practice. What the identification and characterisation of genes does allow, however, is the development of the biology of a disease at a pace that was unparalleled prior to their identification. For instance, it may be possible to create animal models based on transgenic approaches (see below) or to develop a variety of assays for the screening of novel therapeutic compounds. The important point is that the molecular genetic approach affords enormous technical resources allowing rapid progress to be made in studying the individual pathophysiologies of a variety of diseases. Finally, it is worth stressing that although the cloning of a particular gene and its relation to a particular disease will inevitably be easiest for diseases with a large inherited component, the contribution of molecular genetics will be significant for both inherited and non-inherited diseases.

MOLECULAR GENETICS OF SKIN: CASE STUDIES

Lists of diseases and the respective genes are not only dull but are of limited use in understanding the way clinical science is advancing. In the following section several recent advances in the molecular genetics of skin disease are discussed and the strategies that have been used to solve these problems are highlighted. Inevitably, the individual strategies are not carried out in isolation and there are already clear examples, such as with keratin genes and epidermolysis bullosa, where different groups pursuing different approaches have complemented each other's work. Certain diseases, such as psoriasis, are also mentioned, not because there have been outstanding successes in the molecular genetics, but because they are areas in which a large number of research groups are working and, if nothing else, they illustrate the intellectual and technical problems which still have to be surmounted.

RETINOIDS, RETINOIC ACID AND RETINOIC ACID RECEPTORS

It has long been known that vitamin A (retinol) and its derivatives, including retinoic acid, are essential for the development and maintenance of normal epithelia. At the beginning of the century Wolbach and Howe (1925) showed that rats fed diets deficient in vitamin A developed a variety of epithelial abnormalities, predominantly involving the respiratory tract and with the development of squamous metaplasia.

These observations were confirmed, and Fell and Mellanby (1953) showed that chick embryonic skin exposed to excess vitamin A changed to a columnar secretory glandular epithelium. Subsequent work on cultured keratinocytes again showed that vitamin A and its derivatives had profound effects on differentiation, in this case inhibiting the differentiation of keratinocytes. The effects of retinoic acid are not confined to epithelial cells, and effects on the differentiation of embryonal carcinoma cells and promyelocytic cells lines are well documented. While these understandings in basic science were emerging, clinicians were using retinol in the treatment of a variety of cutaneous diseases, although toxicity limited its therapeutic role.

Retinoids have long been known to have an anti-tumour effect, and it was during the screening of compounds for biological activity, using the mouse papilloma assay system, that a number of novel retinoids were identified which were therapeutically more successful than retinol. Today retinoic acid and its derivative etretinate find important roles in the treatment of acne and a variety of dyskeratoses. Retinoids potently inhibit sebum excretion rate, hence their use in acne, and clinically appear to alter the pattern of keratinisation, leading to their use in a variety of dyskeratoses and ichthyotic conditions. Given their therapeutic role, it is therefore natural to ask whether any of these diseases could primarily be due to abnormalities of retinoid metabolism, including end organ resistance to the effects of endogenous retinoids.

The potent effects of retinoids on the differentiation of cells in a variety of different test systems, and the fact that these effects were evident at low drug concentration, suggested that the effects were mediated by specific receptors that interacted with the genome. A family of cytoplasmic receptors, including cellular retinoic acid binding protein (CRABP), had been identified. However, on the basis of sequence information these binding proteins were not thought likely to mediate the putative effects of retinoic acid. Based on biochemical approaches, attempts to clone the putative retinoic acid receptors (RARs) that interacted with the genome have been unsuccessful. The molecular biological approach to this problem relied on various groups whose interest was not so much in retinoic acid biology itself, but in looking at the broader question of how gene transcription and hence protein expression is controlled. A central problem of molecular genetics has been the elucidation of the control of tissue-specific gene expression; keratins are expressed in keratinocytes and not in red cell precursors, whereas globin genes are transcribed in the latter but not in the former. Corticosteroid hormones have been thought to act as gene enhancers, i.e. the hormone plus a receptor binds upstream of particular target genes and switches on or facilitates transcription from that particular gene. In this sense an enhancer can be viewed as a volume control for the output of that gene.

By the mid- and late 1980s a variety of groups had identified such receptors for oestrogen, androgen and thyroid hormones, which together have been grouped as the steroid/thyroid receptor superfamily (Evans, 1988). In a clear example of how the technology drives the subject, these groups screened DNA libraries looking for related DNA sequences which they hoped would code for related receptors. An important heuristic point is that it is the technical facility of molecular genetics, the ability to screen plasmid libraries with one probe, and the ability to alter the conditions of that library screening or library hybridisation in such a way that related rather than identical sequences are picked up, that guided the direction of future work. Two major laboratories identified, within their DNA libraries, sequences which although similar to steroid receptors were not identical (Petkovitch et al., 1987; Giguere et al., 1987). Based on the known structure of the receptors already identified, it was possible to manipulate these newly identified clones to show that not only could they function as enhancers, but that they could bind retinoic acid specifically. So therefore, while at a superficial level the discovery of these RARs could be looked upon as serendipitous, more meaningfully the discovery was the result of an experimental strategy that was biased towards novelty and new discovery.

The discovery of the RARs, and the subsequent discovery that some members of a family of *nuclear* RARs are specifically expressed in skin, has given a major boost to the work on retinoids (Rees, 1992). It is interesting to examine exactly what identification of the genes coding for these receptors now allows clinical scientists to study. Firstly, based on the sequence structure it is possible to generate antibodies to these receptors. Here considerable technical problems still remain, as the antibodies made to date appear to perform poorly on tissue immunocytochemistry. The availability of the cloned DNA means that it is possible to study receptor expression in disease, either using Northern blotting (similar to Southern blotting, only RNA size fractionated rather than DNA and therefore information about gene expression is obtained) and techniques such as *in situ* hybridisation in which individual RNA transcripts coding for particular proteins may be studied in tissue sections. To date, limited studies have been performed using these techniques, but already for the nuclear RARs and the cytoplasmic retinoic binding proteins, abnormalities have been observed in dyskeratotic conditions. Thirdly, of course, as described above, this family of receptors acts as enhancers: it is thought that ligand, probably retinoic acid or its derivatives or metabolites, binds to the receptor inducing conformational change, which allows the receptor–ligand complex to bind upstream of target gene sequences, enhancing transcription from these particular genes. With recombinant DNA technology it is possible to assay this ability by placing particular reporter genes next to DNA sequences that confer specificity to binding of the receptor–ligand complex and to assay a variety of test compounds in transfected cells. Although this procedure sounds formidable, it is relatively straightforward and allows a whole range of novel retinoids developed by the pharmaceutical industry to be rapidly screened for biological activity. So here is an example of where cloning and characterisation of a particular gene, even when its exact mechanism of action is not understood, allows drug development to proceed far more cheaply, far more humanely and far more quickly than was feasible previously.

Finally, does the characterisation and isolation of the RARs allow detailed examination of the molecular genetics of the skin diseases which are treated by retinoic acid or its derivatives? Retinoids are potent therapeutic agents, widely used in the treatment of acne and in a variety of disorders of dyskeratinisation. Is it possible that some of these diseases are due to abnormalities of retinoic acid receptors, and if so, how can they be studied and identified? Although the genomic structure of the RARs appears quite complex, it is possible to use the techniques outlined in an earlier section of this chapter to look for mutations in these receptors. Therefore, if it is believed that RARs, for instance, may be *candidate* genes for a condition such as psoriasis or Darier's disease, then DNA can be extracted from the individual patients, Southern blotted and differences in the size of the fragments compared with normal controls. This technique, relying on the use of RFLPs, is unlikely to yield positive information because of the infrequency of the restriction fragment polymorphisms themselves. However, using the PCR, individual exons of the receptors can be amplified and sequenced, and differences noted between patients with a particular disease and controls. In addition, because the RARs themselves will have an enhancer element lying upstream from the coding region of the gene in the DNA, these sequences can also be amplified and mutations identified which may result in impaired or even over-expression of the receptors. With respect to retinoids, the farthest advanced of these approaches at present is the use of the enhancer assays as a screening test for novel compounds, and to date no clear mutations have been identified to account for any human disease. Nevertheless, the receptors have only been cloned in the last few years and several groups are pursuing these various experimental stategies.

KERATIN GENES, EPIDERMOLYSIS BULLOSA AND TRANSGENIC MICE

Keratins are intermediate filaments characteristic of epithelial tissues (Fuchs, 1988). They are normally expressed in pairs: one acidic keratin with one basic keratin. Skin expresses a particular pattern of keratins, with K5 and K14 in the basal cells, and K1 and K10 in suprabasal cells. Disease states are characterised by aberrant keratin expression, such as is the case in psoriasis, where K6 and K16 are expressed instead of K1 and K10. Keratins are abundantly expressed proteins and it was because of this that they were among some of the first human genes cloned. Following the cloning of some of the keratins, a variety of specific antibodies were raised and used to study keratin gene expression in several diseases. As outlined, psoriasis and other hyperproliferative disorders, including skin tumours, are characterised by abnormal keratin gene expression. Although the first keratin genes were identified in the early 1980s and many studies of keratin gene expression in disease have been carried out, none of these studies identified the function of the keratin molecules and the likely result of mutations in keratin genes. The elucidation of this, on the one hand basic biological problem, and on the other hand explanation of the aetiology of an inherited blistering disorder, has been one of the astonishing success stories of the molecular genetic approach to disease. Intriguingly, different groups using different strategies arrived at the answer almost simultaneously – something which is increasingly common in molecular genetics.

One of the standard approaches to molecular genetics has been that of reverse genetics, or what is now called 'positional cloning' – literally cloning on the basis of the gene's position. Pedigrees of patients with a particular pathological phenotype are identified, linkage analysis is performed with DNA probes that detect polymorphisms in the population, and with considerable luck and work a particular area of the chromosome can be implicated in harbouring the mutant gene associated with the pathological phenotype. It is important to note that, for this strategy to succeed, large pedigrees are helpful, clear and correct clinical diagnosis is essential, and related to the gene, either within it or near it, must be polymorphisms that are informative in the population, i.e. yield useful information about whether recombination has taken place or not. The strategy of reverse genetics or positional cloning has so far been the mainstay of the molecular genetic approach to disease and has notched up a number of striking successes, including the localisation of the gene for cystic fibrosis. Using this approach it was reported that one variant of epidermolysis bullosa simplex, a superficial inherited blistering disease, maps to one of the known positions of human keratin genes and appears to be caused by a mutation in a coding region for one of these proteins. However, while the work was in progress, Elaine Fuchs and her group, who had been interested in keratin biology for many years, reported the results of making mice transgenic for a human keratin gene. Transgenic mice contain a foreign gene which has been inserted into the male pronucleus at conception. These mice may then express the protein coded for by this DNA. In the case of the keratin work, a human keratin gene with a mutation which was expected to abolish the normal function of the protein had been used to raise transgenic progeny. The experiment was a success: soon after birth the transgenic mice developed blisters, particularly at sites of trauma, which mirrored the clinical picture observed in some cases of epidermolysis bullosa (Vassar et al., 1991). Subsequently these workers went on to examine the mice histologically and also patients suffering from epidermolysis bullosa, and confirmed that some variants of the epidermolysis bullosa simplex were the result of mutations in basal cell keratins.

So here are examples of molecular genetic approaches which are complementary – one where the gene of interest is unknown and is identified using positional cloning, and another where the question is the reverse, i.e. 'We have a gene, what is its function?' It is important to note that the two approaches are not exclusive and that mapping a disease to a particular area of the chromosome will perhaps lead to a situation where genes which have already been identified as residing within this area will suggest themselves as candidates for a particular disease phenotype. The use of transgenic mice in understanding human molecular genetics is likely to increase. A related but technically more demanding technique – homologous recombination – allows not just the creation of the mouse in which an additional gene may be expressed (in addition to the mouse's normal alleles) but the replacement of a mouse allele with a recombinant gene such that one of the wild type alleles is no longer evident. This is an extremely powerful investigative tool which, although technically demanding, has found increasing use in studying retinoid biology and, as will be mentioned briefly in a later section, in looking at the effects of developmentally regulated and potentially oncogenic genes.

SKIN CARCINOGENESIS

Although non-melanoma skin cancer is probably the commonest human malignancy, the molecular genetics of skin cancer has received scant attention until very recently. This may in part relate to the relative success of therapies for treating such cancers. Nevertheless, as a model system for understanding human epithelial skin neoplasia, skin is probably unrivalled. Malignancies are common, usually eminently treatable, and a variety of stages of neoplasia from benign epitheliomas through dysplasia and in situ carcinoma to invasive carcinoma with metastasis can be observed and sampled. The bodily distribution of skin neoplasia, together with the known epidemiology, suggests that ultraviolet (UV) light is the main mutagen, and recent evidence has suggested characteristic 'molecular footprints' induced by UV mutation in human skin carcinomas. Skin neoplasia also demonstrates the weakness of a rigid distinction between environmentally caused disease and genetic causes: UV light is the main carcinogen, but as studies of human migration patterns and the world-wide epidemiology of non-melanoma skin cancer clearly demonstrate, the genetic determinants of skin pigmentation are clearly of major importance (Celtic versus non-Celtic Caucasian, or Caucasian versus Negro skin).

Gorlin's syndrome is an autosomal dominantly inherited syndrome character-ised by numerous basal cell carcinomas at a young age, skeletal and endocrine abnormalities, characteristic facial appearance and small pits on the hands. Like so many syndromes, the clinical picture suggests that a single gene can cause abnormalities in a variety of different organ systems, and therefore identifying the gene may not only be of interest in this instance in understanding skin neoplasia, but also in understanding a variety of aspects of morphogenesis. Based on extensive pedigree analysis and using classical positional genetic approaches, two groups have recently localised the syndrome to chromosome 9 (Farndon et al., 1992; Reis et al., 1992). This work illustrates a number of issues relating to the molecular genetics of disease in general.

Firstly, as touched upon earlier, if one is not adopting a candidate gene approach, then to map a disease by positional cloning requires large pedigrees, and frequent polymorphisms throughout the genome are necessary, such that the disease can be related to one of these polymorphisms. Recently, positional cloners have seized upon a strategy which makes use of repeated sequences, the highly polymorphic lengths of non-coding DNA which, as mentioned earlier, are scattered through the genome. The function of these micro-satellite sequences is unknown, but of practical importance is the fact that the lengths of the repeated sequences are highly polymorphic between individuals. This means that once primer sequences outside the polymorphic region are determined, the PCR can be used to amplify these areas of DNA, and because of their polymorphisms these can be used as highly informative markers for linkage analysis.

Secondly, although the chromosomal position of a particular disease may have been mapped, moving from the megabase scale down to the thousands of bases required for sequencing and characterisation of the gene, within the area of a chromosome, is a major undertaking. Fortunately a variety of techniques are now making this work more straightforward. They include pulsed field gel electrophoresis – a form of gel electrophoresis which allows one to resolve DNA fragments measuring hundreds of thousands of bases long – coupled with the ability to clone large pieces of DNA in artificial chromosomes based on yeast chromosomes. Nevertheless, if one were to look at the example of familial polyposis coli, considerable problems would be encountered, some of which would be unpredictable in moving from chromosomal position to identifying the precise gene responsible for an abnormality.

Thirdly, by analogy with familial polyposis coli and ordinary colon cancer, one may ask whether the identification of the gene that causes Gorlin's syndrome, which occurs with an incidence of perhaps one in 80 000 individuals, is going to be relevant to the understanding of the far greater number of tumours occurring in individuals without Gorlin's syndrome. The point here, as with familial polyposis coli, the retinoblastomas and other genes that have been associated with neoplasia, is that insight into the cause of the rare syndromes may provide a better understanding of, say, the basal cell carcinomas occurring in non-Gorlin's patients. For instance, it is quite possible that the particular area of chromosome that is abnormal in Gorlin's syndrome may also be deleted or mutated in basal cell carcinomas occurring in non-Gorlin's patients. There is already preliminary evidence that this may indeed be the case.

Apart from Gorlin's syndrome, a variety of other oncogenes have been identified in non-melanoma skin cancer. For example p53, a tumour suppressor gene (i.e. a gene whose function in the wild type appears to be to suppress malignancy, whereas the mutated form is associated with progression to malignancy), is likely to be involved in a variety of skin neoplasms. The evidence is preliminary at present, but it is likely that p53 mutation contributes to basal cell carcinoma development and squamous cell carcinoma progression, and may indeed mutate at an early stage in the progression to malignancy. Of interest here is the occurrence of a variety of neoplasms in the Li Fraumeni syndrome, which is an inherited syndrome associated with mutation of the p53 gene. Patients with Li Fraumeni syndrome have a variety of neoplasms, including melanoma, but curiously non-melanoma skin cancer is not prominent among their tumours. This may relate to the specific mutation in the p53 in these families or may suggest that other rate-limiting steps are more important in skin carcinogenesis than is the case with some internal malignancies.

Apart from p53, mutations in oncogenes have been relatively difficult to find in skin tumours. A variety of *ras* mutations have been found to be important in the development of neoplasia in mouse skin. In humans there is some evidence that in a minority of tumours *ras* mutations may be important, although relatively little work has been published on this matter. Whatever the putative oncogene, researchers are increasingly using transgenic mice or mice in which homologous recombination has been performed in order to examine the effects of mutated oncogenes. Recently it has been reported that mice in which both copies of the p53 gene have been inactivated by homologous recombination, although developmentally normal, develop a variety of tumours at an early age. Other groups are using transgenic approaches to over-express mutant *ras* genes in mouse skin, resulting in the widespread development of neoplasia. These developments will not only help elucidate the mechanisms of oncogenesis, but offer assay systems in which to develop novel chemotherapeutic agents.

DISORDERS OF PIGMENTATION

WAARDENBURG'S AND SPLOTCH SYNDROMES

As has been discussed above, transgenic approaches and homologous recombination offer many opportunities to use animal genetics to elucidate the pathogenesis of human disease. Frequently, different experimental strategies looking at human disease and animal genetics overlap, such that work in one system suggests work in another. The recent identification of a molecular defect in some cases of Waardenburg's syndrome is such an example (Hill and Van Heyningen, 1992).

Waardenburg's syndrome is a hereditary disease responsible for over 2% of cases of congenital deafness, and is characterised by nerve deafness, a displacement of the inner corner of the eye and piebaldism (piebaldism is defined as a genetic disorder of melanocytes of skin and hair with patchy depigmentation of the skin and a white forelock). Based on homology to genes in *Drosophila melanogaster* which have been known to be responsible for segmentation and segment polarity, mouse (and human) *Pax* genes have been identified. The distribution of *Pax 3* genes during mouse embryogenesis, coupled with the mapping of *Pax 3* to the approximal part of chromosome 1 in the mouse, suggested that mutations in *Pax* may be responsible for the pigmentary abnormalities in a mouse mutant named *Splotch* which are localised to chromosome 1. Sequencing of *Pax 3* in *Splotch* mice confirmed that this was indeed the cause of the phenotypic abnormality. Although there are significant differences, in terms of mapping of known genes, a variety of areas of mouse chromosomes have a clear homologous relationship to large areas of human chromosomes. Type 1 Waardenburg syndrome was mapped to an area of chromosome 2, which is thought to be homologous to an area on chromosome 1 in the mouse where the *Splotch* gene had been located. The overlapping phenotypes and the relationship between the map positions between some cases of Waardenburg's and Splotch suggested that the syndromes could result from defects in homologous genes. Various groups then set about analysing the human homologue of *Pax 3* (called *HuP2*) and were able to confirm that mutations in this gene are the cause of some cases of Waardenburg's syndrome. This work clearly demonstrates the interplay between animal and human work, and the interaction between positional cloning and candidate gene approaches. Not only is the molecular basis of the disease now more apparent, but the *Splotch* mouse may well be useful as a model of Waardenburg's syndrome on which to test therapeutic agents, and further understanding of the morphogenic abnormalities.

ALBINISM

Ocular cutaneous albinism is a group of genetic disorders of melanocytes resulting in reduced or absent melanisation in skin and the eyes. Judging by the frequency of pigmentary abnormalities in a wide variety of genetic disorders, situated on several different chromosomes, man may be like mice, in that a large number of genes (over 50 in the mouse) control hair colour. As with Waardenburg's syndrome discussed above, this opens up several molecular genetic approaches which can exploit the excellent mapping facilities that mice afford, together with a large number of mutants from which to characterise genes and then to search for human homologues which may account for cases of albinism. Using this approach, a variety of genes which may share sequence homology with each other within the mouse can be used to identify genes in humans. This approach has revealed a large number of mutations in the tyrosinase gene (Kikuchi *et al.*, 1990), one of the major enzymes involved in melanin formation accounting for a number of different types of ocular cutaneous albinism. As more loci related to mutations in mice are characterised, the possibilities increase for using these gene probes to study those genetic abnormalities in humans where pigmentary abnormalities are part of the syndrome but not the primary abnormality. Information about primarily non-cutaneous disease may therefore be obtained.

MOLECULAR GENETICS OF PSORIASIS

Psoriasis is an inflammatory scaly dermatosis with a fluctuating course. It affects up to 2% of most populations. The frequency of the condition, together with its familial nature and the higher concordance among monozygotic twins compared with dizygotic twins, all suggest that molecular genetic approaches to the aetiology of psoriasis may be fruitful. Nevertheless, despite these apparent attractions, a variety of problems stand in the way of cloning a putative psoriasis gene by positional cloning methods, and therefore alternative strategies may be more successful.

Although psoriasis is clearly familial, the nature of the inheritance is unclear. Sex linkage can be excluded because of the equal incidence among the sexes; a simple autosomal recessive or autosomal dominant mode of inheritance with complete penetrance will, however, not explain the observed familial nature. The necessity for two alleles (recessive) at each of two unlinked loci or an autosomal dominant with a penetrance of 0.4–0.7 would, however, explain the observed familial pattern. Incomplete penetrance, which in itself causes considerable difficulty for positional cloning approaches, is compounded by the possibility of genetic heterogeneity among psoriatics, particularly with respect to certain HLA types, such as Cw6. Also, the age of the onset of the disease is so varied that it may manifest itself for the first time in an 80-year-old; in fact onset over 100 years of age has been recorded! The fact that the disease can appear in the elderly, coupled with the wide variation in the severity of the symptoms, means that assignment of an individual within a pedigree to a particular phenotype may be impossible. Most diseases for which genes have been successfully identified by positional cloning are characterised by a clear pattern of inheritance and clear diagnostic criteria. Nevertheless, a variety of approaches other than positional cloning have been undertaken. Candidate genes, perhaps RARs, since retinoids are used as therapeutic agents in the management of psoriasis, may be important. Certain subgroups of psoriatics have an association with HLA B27, and transgenic mice expressing human HLA B27 have been noted to develop cutaneous and joint abnormalities at least reminiscent of psoriasis and psoriatic arthropathy. Alternatively, a variety of cytokine abnormalities have been described in psoriasis, including over-expression of transforming growth factor α (TGFα) in the epidermis. Recently mice transgenic for TGFα have been produced and, although they show cutaneous abnormalities including acanthosis, the inflammatory component does not match that seen in psoriasis. As more and more cytokine abnormalities are described in psoriasis, it is likely that these sorts of approaches will continue.

CONCLUSION

It is just over 10 years since the first human genes were cloned and characterised. The rate of progress and the achievement of the molecular genetic approach have been considerable. If the number of genes identified and sequenced is plotted, the line is logarithmic with respect to time rather than linear. As more of the genes coding for the structural proteins of the epidermis and dermis are characterised, it seems likely that many cases of ichthyosis and epidermolysis bullosa will be found to be secondary to mutations in keratin or collagen genes. These are astonishing developments. Nevertheless, a major challenge for the molecular genetic approach to skin disease lies in developing experimental strategies that will allow the study of the major inflammatory disorders that make up much of dermatological practice. In these instances, identification of the gene responsible, for example an inflammatory mediator, is only the first step in creating a biology that will allow the prediction of the course of clinical events and therapeutic intervention. Treatment of the majority of cutaneous diseases will remain pharmacological, but the pharmacological approach to therapy will itself be increasingly dominated by the strategies of molecular genetics.

REFERENCES

Evans RM (1988). The steroid and thyroid hormone receptor superfamily. *Science* **240**, 889–895.

Farndon PA, Del Mastro RG, Evans DGR and Kilpatrick MW (1992) Location of gene for Gorlin syndrome. *Lancet* **339**, 581–582.

Fell H and Mellanby E (1953) Metaplasia produced in cultures of chick ectoderm by high vitamin A. *Journal of Physiology* **119**, 470–488.

Fuchs E (1988) Keratins as biochemical markers of epithelial differentiation. *Trends in Genetics* **4**, 277–281.

Giguere V, Ong E, Segui P and Evans R (1987) Identification of a receptor for the morphogen retinoic acid. *Nature* **330**, 624–629.

Hill R and Van Heyningen V (1992) Mouse mutations and human disorders are paired. *Trends in Genetics* **8**, 4.

Kikuchi H, Hara S, Ishiguro S, Tamai M and Watanabe M (1990) Detection of point mutation in the tyrosinase gene of a Japanese albino patient by a direct sequencing of amplified DNA. *Human Genetics* **85**, 123–124.

Petkovitch M, Brand N, Krust A and Chambon P (1987) A human retinoic acid receptor which belongs to the family of nuclear receptors. *Nature* **330**, 444–450.

Rees J (1992) The molecular biology of retinoic acid receptors: orphan from good family seeks home. *British Journal of Dermatology* **126**, 97–104.

Reis A, Kuster W, Gebel E, Fuhrmann W, Groth W, Kuklik M, Wegner RD, Linss G, Hamm H, Wolff G, Gustafson G, Burger J and Neitzel H (1992) Localisation of gene for the naevoid basal-cell carcinoma syndrome. *Lancet* **339**, 617.

Vassar R, Coulombe P, Degenstein L, Albers R and Fuchs E (1991) Mutant keratin expression in transgenic mice causes marked abnormalities resembling a human genetic disease. *Cell* **64**, 365–380.

Wolbach S and Howe P (1925) Tissue changes following deprivation of fat soluble A vitamin. *Journal of Experimental Medicine* **42**, 753–778.

FURTHER READING

Emery AEH and Mueller RF (1988) *Student Notes. Elements of Medical Genetics*, 7th edn. Edinburgh: Churchill Livingstone.

Watson JD, Gilman M, Witkowski J and Zoller M (1992) *Recombinant DNA*, 2nd edn. New York: WH Freeman.

Weatherall DJ (1991) *The New Genetics and Clinical Practice*, 3rd edn. Oxford: Oxford University Press.

10 Medicinal Chemistry in Dermatology

BRAHAM SHROOT

This chapter outlines the basic principles of medicinal chemistry and illustrates with selected examples how this discipline can be applied to therapeutics in dermatology. A concise description of the structure of the skin, as the target of the selected drugs, is given in order to better appreciate its cellular pharmacology. Notions of barrier function are described to illustrate some aspects of drug delivery. Drug action and its relationship to chemical structure will be exemplified in three sections from the fields of steroids, retinoids and finally dithranol (anthralin).

INTRODUCTION

To a large extent, drug discovery is serendipitous and the tasks of drug hunters engaged in the search for new and improved therapies are complex. This is obvious when we consider each of the following five key disciplines which make up the discovery and development processes:

Pharmaceutics
Pharmacokinetics
Pharmacodynamics
Toxicology
Human safety and efficacy

In the space available it would be impossible to describe each discipline in detail, but we can introduce the reader to a limited number of significant points within the context of the chapter.

Firstly, pharmaceutics concerns the drug substance itself or *active principle* and its vehicle or *formulation*. The study of this process assumes that chemical identity, purity and stability of the active principle are well defined, and that when the substance is presented in a formulation suitable for the proposed use the stability of the product is defined from both chemical and rheological standpoints. The physico-chemical properties of the active substance, its physical state (solution, suspension, particle size) and its concentration in the

Molecular Aspects of Dermatology. Edited by G.C. Priestley.
© 1993 by John Wiley & Sons Ltd

vehicle govern the effectiveness of the treatment. In addition, for topical therapy, other factors such as patient compliance and the nature of the skin lesion are influenced by the art and skill of the formulator and are often described as cosmetic acceptability. Lastly, the skin has also been viewed as a port of entry for drugs acting systemically and thus the nature of the delivery system employed will be different again.

Pharmacokinetics covers absorption, distribution, metabolism and excretion of the active substance from its formulation. Recently this area has become the subject of intense research, in view of the trend in modern drug research to regard the body as a series of compartments. Thus the efficacy of drugs in relation to their concentration at the site of action, as well as their presence as a potential toxicological risk in other organs, is now studied. Similarly, the identity of metabolites has become the subject of much attention, now extending to the search for optical isomers, because these isomers can have different pharmacological and toxicological properties from the parent drug (Williams, 1985). This observation stems from the stereospecific nature of many receptor-mediated processes.

Although they have the same chemical properties, stereoisomers of the active principle have mirror image configurations in space which may result in different affinities for target proteins and consequently dictate different biological actions. This last point leads to the notion of receptor-mediated drug action. No matter how attractive this idea may be to the pharmacologist or chemist, it must be stressed at the outset that the concept helps us understand, but does not fully explain, the mode of action of drugs. We have come a long way from Ehrlich's simple lock-and-key description of a ligand and its receptor, but the basic chemical and biochemical principles remain the same. Today we argue more in terms of the nature of the molecular interactions surrounding the docking of such entities and have realised that, in many cases, the resulting complex itself acts as a ligand for other proteins or target sequences on DNA or chromatin. Not only is the primary amino acid sequence of proteins important, but also pertinent is the secondary and tertiary structure, related to protein folding. Before knowing the nature of the molecular targets, the identity and location of the target cell are primary considerations in drug action and design and therefore a simplified description of the skin as a target organ for drugs is appropriate here. It must be stressed that although this information is useful, little is known about the structure and function of the *abnormal* cell in the diseased state treated by the drugs described below. Application of techniques such as *in situ* hybridisation and the use of reconstructed skin *in vitro* will shed light on these questions in the near future.

THE SKIN

The skin is a multicellular organ comprising three distinct major compartments. It has a blood and nerve supply adapted to the proximity of the organ to the external environment as well as to its own physiological needs. The skin also contains many related appendages, some of which have openings to the surface, such as the pilosebaceous units and eccrine sweat glands. These appendages have their own specific cellular composition relating to their function. Figure 10.1 shows the cellular composition of the skin.

The deepest compartment, the *hypodermis*, consists mainly of adipocytes and besides being a source of energy and providing insulation and mechanical protection it also serves to store lipophilic substances. The hair bulb is located at this level. The *dermis*, the intermediate compartment, contains fibroblasts which manufacture an extracellular matrix consisting of insoluble fibrous proteins such as collagen and elastin. This matrix houses the complex network of nerves and blood vessels supplying the skin, and also maintains its elasticity. The extracellular matrix is made up of polysaccharides and glycosoamino-glycans such as hyaluronic acid and dermatan sulphate. As will be seen later, the constituents of the extracellular matrix are a target for drugs which reverse photo-induced damage. In addition, the fibroblast is thought to play a major role in communication between the dermis and the epidermis by secreting signal molecules. The dermis, which is between 500 and 1000 μm thick, also contains the sebaceous glands. These organelles are also a target for drugs but their accessibility is impaired by dilution after percutaneous application. The dermis and the epidermis are separated by a basement membrane, the nature of which is the subject of intense research (see Chapter 4).

By far the most-studied compartment of the skin is the *epidermis.* This multilayered epithelium, 100 μm thick, contains three main cell types: the keratinocyte, the melanocyte and the Langerhans cell (Fig. 10.1). It was previously thought that the sole function of the keratinocyte was to terminally differentiate as it migrated from the basement membrane (basal cells) to the outermost *corneocyte* (horny) layer. The corneocyte, being an anucleate insoluble structure, serves as a part of the protective barrier to the external environment by forming a multilayered graphite-like matrix.

Corneocytes are held together by a complex mixture of simple and complex lipids, water and other substances which are chemically undefined. The structure of the horny layer (see Fig. 10.1) was described by Elias in terms of a 'bricks and mortar' model, which has been used by biochemists to try to understand the barrier function of the epidermis (Elias, 1983). Although convenient, this view of the epidermis has been modified because it ignored the factor of time. The transit time from the basal layer to the horny layer is about 1 month in normal skin, yet after mild injury (tape stripping) or major trauma (psoriasis) turnover time is considerably shortened and in addition the nature and distribution pattern of skin lipids change markedly. It is now widely accepted that the horny layer is dynamic and that it can adapt rapidly to minor changes in its environment. Recent studies show that there are specific lipids bound covalently to the corneocytes (Wertz *et al.*, 1989) and also that enzymes situated just beneath the horny layer regulate the function of specific adherence proteins. Interplay of these systems with drugs and their vehicles can lead to

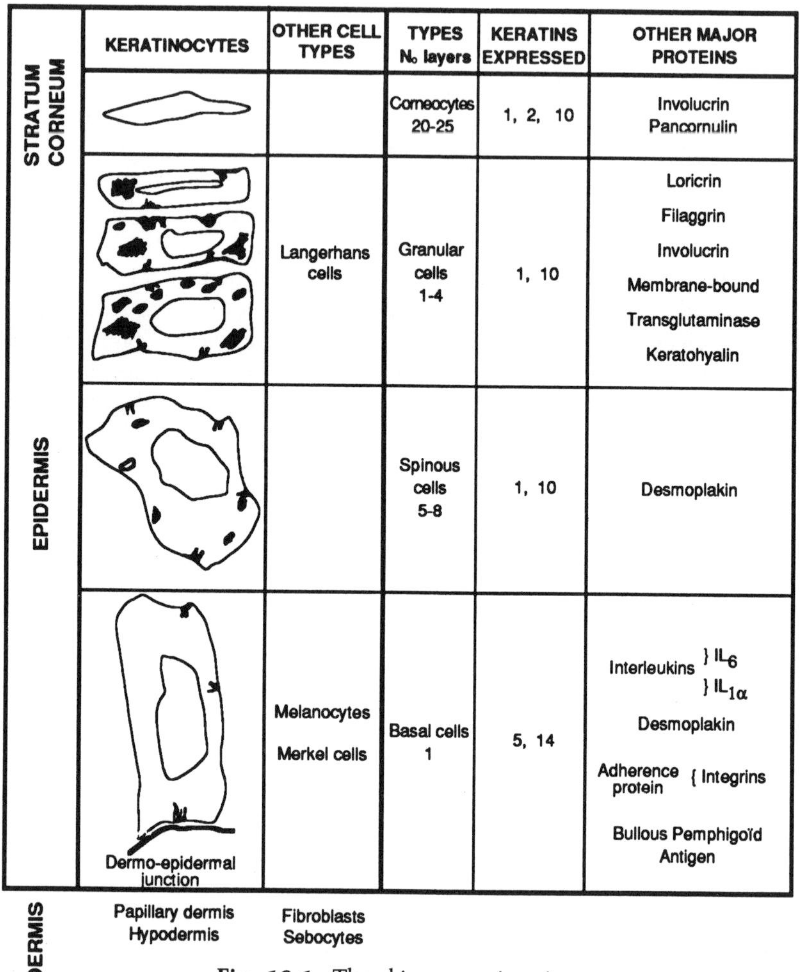

	KERATINOCYTES	OTHER CELL TYPES	TYPES No. layers	KERATINS EXPRESSED	OTHER MAJOR PROTEINS
STRATUM CORNEUM			Corneocytes 20-25	1, 2, 10	Involucrin Pancornulin
EPIDERMIS		Langerhans cells	Granular cells 1-4	1, 10	Loricrin Filaggrin Involucrin Membrane-bound Transglutaminase Keratohyalin
			Spinous cells 5-8	1, 10	Desmoplakin
		Melanocytes Merkel cells	Basal cells 1	5, 14	Interleukins } IL_6 } $IL_{1\alpha}$ Desmoplakin Adherence protein { Integrins Bullous Pemphigoïd Antigen
	Dermo-epidermal junction				
DERMIS	Papillary dermis Hypodermis	Fibroblasts Sebocytes			

Fig. 10.1. The skin: a concise view

local side-effects, such as irritation, or to alteration of barrier function.

The second major discovery concerning the epidermis, and the keratinocyte in particular, was that epidermal cells can produce cytokines following stimulation. The possibility exists that antigen-presenting Langerhans cells can act as a shuttle from the skin to the lymphatic system, or trigger the appearance of activated T-lymphocytes in the epidermis and this has opened the door to the study of the immunological function of the epidermis. Thus the simple role of the keratinocyte as a keratin-producing component of stratified epithelium is now expanded into a key part of the body's early immunological responses. This of course has profound consequences for the action of drugs in the skin, in that what was formerly regarded as antiproliferative action, or modulation of cellular differentiation, must now be re-interpreted in terms of more elaborate

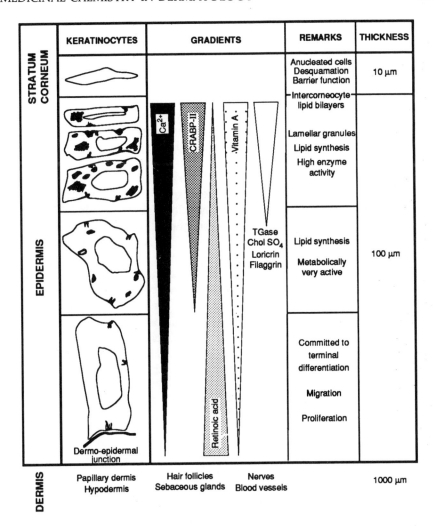

mechanisms. A caveat to this, however, is that some immunosuppressive drugs, such as cyclosporin, which are effective in the treatment of severe psoriasis by the systemic route, are ineffective topically.

CORTICOSTEROIDS

STEROIDAL ANTI-INFLAMMATORY DRUGS

Clinical indications: Inflammatory dermatoses mainly psoriasis, atopic and contact eczema.

Local side-effects: Atrophy of the epidermis and dermis, irritation and impairment of would healing.

Systemic side-effects: Suppression of adrenocorticoid function (decreased levels of plasma cortisol).

Mode of action

The locally acting steroids work in a non-specific manner. Their effects are multiple and occur at most levels of cell function. Figure 10.2 summarises these effects. One pathway involves acting on the synthesis of proteins such as lipocortin, which inhibits phospholipase A_2. This enzyme in turn controls the supply of arachidonic acid, which on oxidation by lipoxygenases or prostaglandin synthetases furnishes mediators of inflammation in the injured cell. By this mechanism steroids could exercise an anti-inflammatory action, if indeed over-expression of lipocortin is associated with chronic inflammation. However, steroids also affect the synthesis of other proteins and interact with other major biochemical pathways (Fig. 10.2). It is almost certain that these drugs act via several such mechanisms. As most cells possess the cytosolic steroid-binding protein, which is believed to transport the ligand to the nucleus where protein transcription is modulated, the challenge in understanding steroid action lies in identifying the target cells. A key feature of the pharmacology of steroids is their vasoconstrictor activity. This shows as a blanching effect on the skin developing 6–9 hours after topical application. A link between this action and steroid potency is widely accepted and has resulted in a classification system ranking these drugs on a scale from I to IV (Stoughton, 1992).

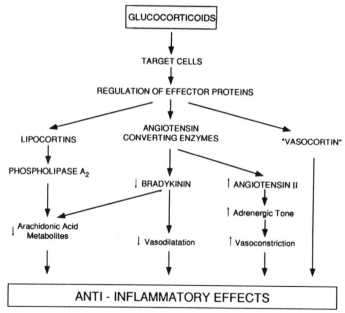

Fig. 10.2. Mode of action of corticosteroids

Table 10.1 lists representative corticosteroids and it is remarkable that betamethasone dipropionate can appear in different categories depending on its formulation (see Table 10.2). This arises because the vehicle can markedly influence the activity of the drug. Occlusive ointments, or vehicles containing penetration enhancers such as propylene glycol, will favour increased concentration of the drug in the deeper skin compartments. When we extrapolate these observations back to the cellular level we might suspect a relationship between the affinity of the steroids for their specific binding proteins and their biological action or their physico-chemical properties. But in general the literature does not support this idea. Within chemically similar series, however, encouraging trends have been identified, and consequently

Table 10.1. Corticosteroid classification

Very strong activity (Class I)	
Clobetasol propionate	0.05%
Betamethasone-17,21-dipropionate	0.05%
with propylene glycol	
Strong activity (Class II)	
Hydrocortisone (butyrate)	0.1%
Betamethasone-17-valerate	0.1% (Class III at 0.05%)
Betamethasone-17,21-dipropionate	0.05%
Desoximethasone	0.25%
Fluocinonide	0.05%, 0.025% (Class III at 0.01%)
Halcinonide	0.1%
Moderate activity (Class III)	
Desonide	0.1%, 0.05%
Fluocortolone–caproate–pivalate	0.5%
Fluocinolone acetonide	0.01%, 0.05% (Class II – ointment)
Flumethasone pivalate	0.02%
Triamcinolone acetonide	0.1%
Triamcinolone benetonide	0.075%
Weak activity (Class IV)	
Hydrocortisone	0.5% and 1%
Methylprednisolone (acetate)	0.25%
Dexamethasone (phosphate)	0.05%

Table 10.2. Influence of the formulation on the potency of betamethasone dipropionate (0.05%)

Formulation	Potency class	
Solution	IV	Weak
Cream	III	
Ointment	II	
Ointment with propylene glycol	I	Very potent

this poses the question of whether corticosteroids should be considered as a single class of drugs.

Substances with the basic tetracyclic structure of the corticosteroids can possess two types of pharmacological action: *glucocorticoid*, with anti-inflammatory activity; and *mineralocorticoid*, acting on the sodium retention and potassium diuresis of the organism. The naturally occurring glucocortico-steroids, such as hydrocortisone, are characterised by the presence of an oxygen function on carbon 11. In Fig. 10.3(a) three endogenous substances are illustrated and the accepted carbon numbering is depicted on the structure of corticosterone. In their attempts to improve beneficial activity in this class of drugs medicinal chemists and pharmacologists use the concept of the *therapeutic index* (TI). This is the ratio of the dose of a given substance provoking toxicity to the pharmacologically effective dose. Ideally, this ratio should be determined in the same species, by the same route and expressed in the same units. Unfortunately a systematic study of therapeutic index by the

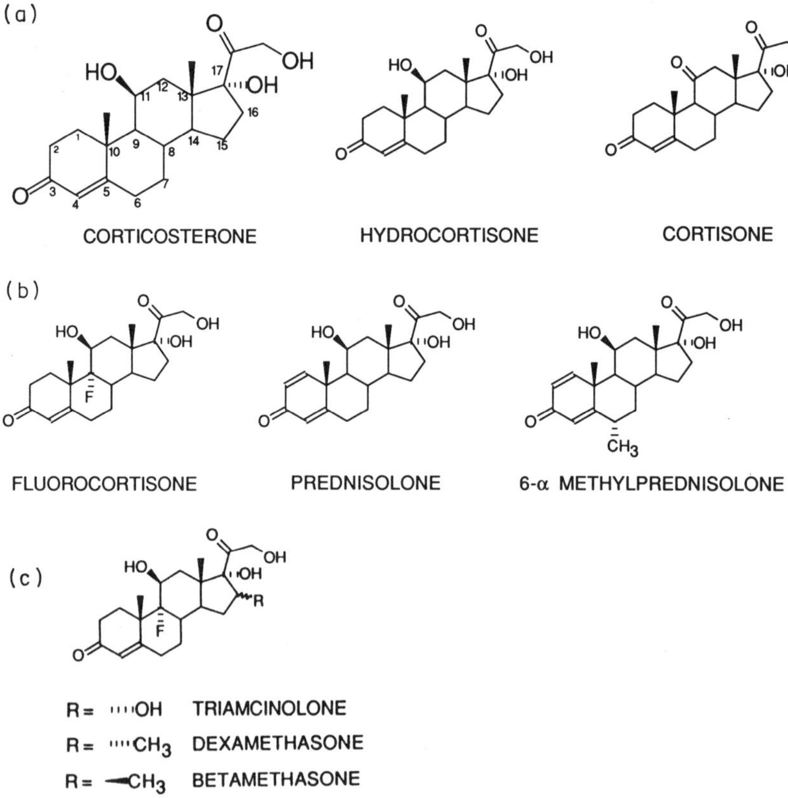

(a)

CORTICOSTERONE   HYDROCORTISONE   CORTISONE

(b)

FLUOROCORTISONE   PREDNISOLONE   6-α METHYLPREDNISOLONE

(c)

R = ''''OH   TRIAMCINOLONE
R = ''''CH$_3$ DEXAMETHASONE
R = —CH$_3$ BETAMETHASONE

Fig. 10.3.

Table 10.3. Therapeutic indices for different corticosteroids

Substance	TI
Hydrocortisone	1.0
Corticosterone	0.02
Desoxycorticosterone	$\ll 0.1$
Fluorocorticosterone	0.1
Prednisolone	5
6α-methylprednisolone	10
Triamcinolone	> 10
Dexamethasone	$\gg 10$
Betamethasone	$\gg 10$

TI = half-maximum dose inducing sodium retention/half-maximum anti-inflammatory dose.

topical route has not been carried out for the corticosteroids. In order to identify compounds with pronounced glucocorticoid rather than mineralocorticoid activity, reference is made below to systemic studies in which the half-maximal dose inducing sodium retention (LD_{50}), will be compared to the half-maximal anti-inflammatory dose (ED_{50}).

Introduction of a fluorine atom at carbon 9 (Fig. 10.3(b), fluorocortisone) markedly increases anti-inflammatory activity but also increases sodium retention, the TI being less than that of hydrocortisone. Introduction of a second double bond in the A ring between carbons 1 and 2 also increases anti-inflammatory activity but the toxicity is reduced, thus giving rise to the success of the prednisolone family (Fig. 10.3(b)). Recently introduced corticosteroids, such as triamcinolone, dexamethasone and betamethasone (Fig. 10.3(c)) have much less mineralocorticoid activity and possess potent anti-inflammatory properties. However, these substances are not devoid of other side-effects such as causing loss of skin collagen (*skin atrophy*), telangiectasia and facial rosacea or, on prolonged application under occlusion, suppression of adrenocortical function.

Since the first therapeutic use of topical hydrocortisone in 1952 by Sultzberger and Witten, the pharmaceutical industry has made a considerable effort to find more potent and less atrophogenic steroids. Table 10.1, listing products by class, shows the wide choice available to the dermatologist. A considerable amount of data exists but care must be taken in extrapolating from cell culture to animals and from animals to man. As indicated earlier, the human skin-blanching assay provides a measure of steroid potency. This test has been carefully documented so that inter-investigator variations are minimised. Extensive use of non-invasive technology has improved quantification of the blanching and thinning phenomena, and considerable validation studies are under way to replace the simple visual and caliper measurements.

The interesting concept of 'soft drugs' has been applied to the corticosteroid family. This concept, devised by Bodor (1984), is based on the premise that drugs can be designed that are extensively metabolised in the body to biologically inactive products. Thus the incorporation of metabolically reactive weak bonds in the structure of a substance can cause it to be deactivated *in vivo* after completing its therapeutic action. This notion is particularly attractive for skin pharmacology in that the target organ is directly in contact with the parent substance and systemic deactivation occurs after transdermal passage. Bodor's idea centred on the metabolism of hydrocortisone to cortenic acid via oxidative decarboxylation of the side chain on carbon 17 (Fig. 10.4a). Thus he sought cortenic acid derivatives which had intrinsic anti-inflammatory activity but which could be metabolically converted to cortenic acid. This was achieved by preparing the disubstituted cortenic acids shown in Fig. 10.4.b

Increasing the lipophilicity of steroids could influence their percutaneous absorption properties. This is the case within well-defined subgroups of compounds, but generalisation of such processes must be made cautiously because different skin sites have different absorption properties (Maibach *et al.*, 1971). This extensive site variation is not always considered when comparing one study with another. A second complication in such comparisons is the chemical and metabolic transformation which may occur in the skin.

To conclude this section, it is clear that corticosteroids have had, and will continue to have, a major place in the topical therapy of inflammatory dermatoses. The search for higher safety margins will proceed through the design of new molecules and better control of the delivery and targeting by formulation research.

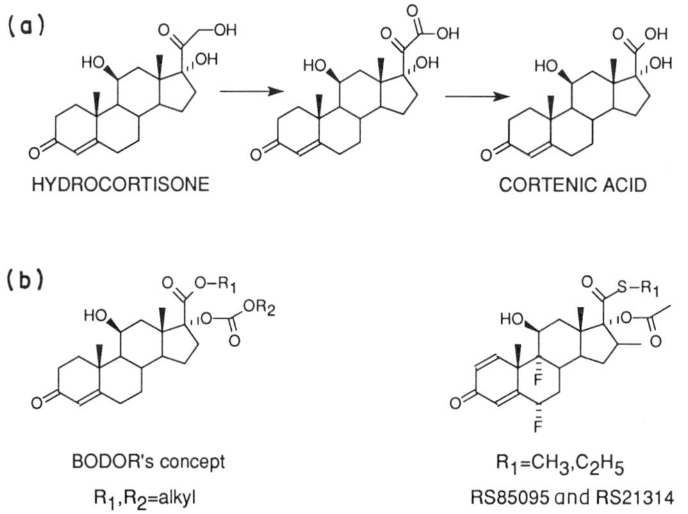

(a)

HYDROCORTISONE   CORTENIC ACID

(b)

BODOR's concept
R_1, R_2 = alkyl

$R_1 = CH_3, C_2H_5$
RS85095 and RS21314

Fig. 10.4.

RETINOIDS

Clinical indications: Acne, psoriasis, photo-induced damage, disorders of keratinisation.

Local side-effects: Erythema, dryness, scaling.

Systemic side-effects: Teratogenicity, bone fragility, chelitis.

It was known over 60 years ago that retinoids, which originate from β-carotene, provoke cutaneous changes, and the therapeutic use of vitamin A in acne was documented in 1943 by J.V. Straumfjord. The history of the clinical use of retinoids, and specifically of retinoic acid, has been described (Stüttgen, 1986). In recent years a more basic role for retinoic acid and its metabolites has been proposed, namely as a morphogen (Eichele and Thaller, 1987). This implies that a lipophilic unsaturated fatty acid of low molecular weight could control embryonic development in a time- and space-dependent manner. Although direct control by retinoic acid in this context has been questioned, its involvement in cellular signal trafficking remains unchallenged. Consequently the means by which the body controls local concentration of retinoic acid, and of its precursors or metabolites, have become focus points for research by workers in many scientific disciplines. This preamble serves the dual purpose of indicating the biological significance of retinoids and the toxic consequences of overdosing, especially in the developing embryo. Essentially, the challenge to the pharmacologist, medicinal chemist and clinician is to improve the low therapeutic ratio associated with retinoids.

A brief description of the retinoids currently used in dermatology will set the scene for a discussion of the current research endeavours. Retinoids are used systematically and topically; different analogues have different therapeutic uses. Only the retinoic acid metabolite 13-*cis*-retinoic acid can be used effectively by both routes, the oral form for severe recalcitrant acne and the topical form for milder forms of the disease. The first 'non-natural' derivative to be developed was the aromatic etretinate, later superseded by the corresponding acid, acitretin. These latter substances, given orally, are prescribed for the treatment of psoriasis, especially pustular psoriasis and mainly when the patient's disease resists other therapy. The concept behind this is that retinoic acid is metabolised and deactivated by oxidation in the cyclohexenyl lipophilic ring portion of the molecule (Fig. 10.5) and aromatisation of this portion would lead to longer-acting substances. This is indeed the case, but the therapeutic ratio is hardly improved (Klaus *et al.*, 1983). A widely used member of the family is all-*trans*-retinoic acid, which has the generic name tretinoin. This substance is approved for topical use in acne and disorders of keratinisation. In addition there are numerous reports of the treatment of photo-induced skin damage and the precancerous condition actinic keratosis (Kligman *et al.*, 1986).

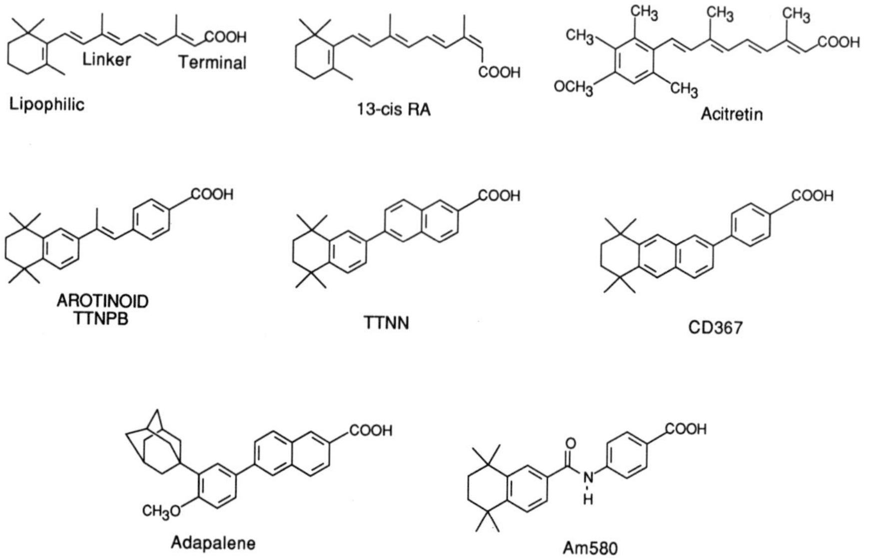

Fig. 10.5.

Table 10.4 lists the therapeutic indices of three families of retinoic acid analogues. As was the case with corticosteroids, there is no report in the literature of studies by topical application in the same species. The indices shown in the table are calculated by comparing the minimal dose inducing hypervitaminosis A syndrome with the dose producing 50% inhibition of cutaneous papillomas in mice treated with the tumour promoter dimethylbenzanthracene. In essence, the structural changes made in the retinoic acid skeleton in two of its three domains, namely the lipophilic and linker regions (Fig. 10.5), do not markedly influence the therapeutic index. Recent data indicate that changes in the carboxylic region produce major improvements in this index. Arotinoid ethyl sulphone causes fewer side-effects than its carboxylic acid equivalent arotinoid acid (Fig. 10.5: the COOH group of arotinoid is replaced by $-SO_2C_2H_5$). This may be a case of a pro-drug, which unlike the soft drug concept described earlier, is activated rather than deactivated *in vivo*. In this

Table 10.4. Therapeutic indices for different retinoids

Substance	TI
All-*trans*-retinoic acid	0.2
13-*cis*-retinoic acid	0.5
Etretinate	2.0
Arotinoid ethyl sulphone	1.0

TI = therapeutic index, defined as the ratio between the minimal dose inducing hypervitaminosis A syndrome and the dose producing 50% inhibition of cutaneous papillomas in mice.

instance the ethyl sulphone group would be converted to a sulphonic acid. The degree of conversion depends on the route, the species and the exposure time. The sulphone form has no retinoid binding characteristics as far as cytosolic and nuclear binding proteins are concerned. Alternatively, it is possible that the sulphone itself acts topically by a mechanism other than that followed by classical retinoids (Klaus *et al.*, 1983).

The milder symptoms of hypervitaminosis A such as chelitis, dry skin, and the more severe effects such as hair loss or bone fragility, are discomforting, but in the main reversible. Thus, careful monitoring of patients on systemic retinoid therapy should avoid major adverse events in the non-gestating patient. In contrast, systemic retinoids must *not* be used by pregnant women: teratogenicity is the most serious side-effect of 13-*cis*-retinoic acid in humans. Full discussion of this subject is outside the scope of this chapter but teratogenicity is a major obstacle in the achievement of the full clinical potential of retinoids or related drugs. The complexity is highlighted by the fact that 13-*cis*- and all-*trans*-retinoic acid are interconvertible *in vivo*, and that in animal species the all-*trans* form is more teratogenic than its isomer. Finally some of the other metabolites (4-oxo) are also highly teratogenic, whereas the glucuronide conjugates are not.

In order to identify new retinoids with a better safety margin, a pharmacological screening programme should include assessment of embryotoxic potential as well as the ability to control cellular differentiation and proliferation (Shroot, 1989). Such a strategy will be illustrated for a structure–activity study of all-*trans*-retinoic acid. A brief description of the well-defined test systems used will be followed by comments on the structures selected. Finally some remarks on the affinity for the key substances to the nuclear and cytosolic retinoic acid-binding proteins will be added.

One well-documented *in vitro* test system for quantifying retinoid activity uses the mouse teratocarcinoma cell line F9. When exposed to micromolar concentrations of retinoids, pronounced morphological changes occur, provoking these cells to revert to their original endodermal phenotype. This change is accompanied by increased secretion of the enzyme plasminogen activator. Thus comparison of the doses producing half-maximal induction of plasminogen activator will define a rank order of potency. Similar, but not identical, ranking can be determined using another assay in cultures of normal human keratinocytes. Measurement of the repression of the membrane-associated transglutaminase (TGase K) by ELISA (enzyme-linked immunosorbent assay) gives a sensitive and rapid assessment of retinoid activity. This enzyme cross-links proteins to an insoluble corneocyte envelope by forming $\varepsilon(\gamma$-glutamyl)-lysine isopeptide bonds. Table 10.5 illustrates the rank potency of some representative retinoic acid analogues in these test systems.

In vivo, the pharmacological action of retinoids on the skin of the *rhino* mouse is well documented. The skin of this mutant has many large and keratin-filled cysts called utricles, which have been compared to the open

Table 10.5. Pharmacology of topical retinoids

Compound	F9[a] (nM)	TGase[b] (nM)	Rhino mouse[c]		
			Comedones	Thickness	r
All-*trans*-retinoic acid	200	11.5	25	55	1.9
13-*cis*-retinoic acid	180	2.6	35	46	1.9
Acitretin	73	12.6	47	45	1.4
Adapalene	45	0.82	43	35	1.1

[a]Concentration of the retinoid producing half-maximal induction of plasminogen activator in the murine teratocarcinoma cell line (F9).
[b]Concentration of the retinoid producing a 50% inhibition of the induction of transglutaminase in normal human keratinocytes *in vitro*.
[c]Animals were treated topically with 0.1% suspension of the drug in acetone for 3 weeks.
Comedones: number of epidermal comedones per centimetre.
Thickness: epidermal thickness in micrometres.
r: measure of the shape and size of the comedone. Values greater than 1 signify comedones being expelled; values less than 1 signify unmodified comedones.

comedones of human acne. By both topical and oral routes retinoids induce changes in the epidermis resulting in a transition from a keratin-packed utricle to a smooth surface. Besides resolution of the utricles, various degrees of hyperplasia can be induced by these substances. By use of image analysis techniques, retinoid effects can be quantified and their rank order of potency can be determined. The vehicle effects noted for steroids are known here too. The ability of this model to discriminate between formulations and even different doses is limited, however, due to the multiple application protocol and saturation of the pharmacological effects.

Teratogenicity is the key factor to assess in the retinoid field. Use of *in vitro* (rat embryo culture) and *in vivo* (mouse limb bud) models helps in the evaluation of such risks.

A brief account of the evolution of retinoid pharmacology and chemistry based on such models will now be given. The activities of the reference substances all-*trans*-retinoic acid, 13-*cis*-retinoic acid, etretinate, acitretin and arotinoid acid will be compared with those of some more recent derivatives whose design and synthesis were early attempts to enhance metabolic and chemical stability. Eventually, a more pronounced departure from the double bond linker array led to the naphthalene TTNN, the stable anthracene CD 367 and amides such as Am 580. If we compare these chemical structures with those of the open double bond variety, the similarity is not obvious. In addition, there is a wide range of potencies among these substances in the test systems. Each of them can be chemically modified, giving rise to a large number of interesting new retinoids some of which, for example adapalene, are undergoing pharmaceutical development.

A major new interest in retinoic acid centres around its action in skin conditions other than acne. One example is the effect of retinoic acid applied topically for 10 weeks to photo-damaged skin. A dermal repair zone was observed in *skh* mice previously irradiated for 10 weeks with UVB light, and there is evidence that retinoic acid can indeed induce the synthesis of new collagen in mice. Although extrapolation of this finding to humans is debatable, it has been shown that prolonged application of tretinoin can repair photo-induced damage to human skin, resulting in the smoothing out of fine wrinkles (Kligman *et al.*, 1986).

In this final section on retinoids, some comments on another approach to drug design will be made. Figure 10.6(a) represents a proposed mode of action of retinoic acid. At the level of the nucleus the retinoids, in particular retinoic acid, act via a specific set of ligand-dependent transactivating proteins – the retinoic acid receptors (RARs) – which are considered to be members of the steroid thyroid superfamily since they share a high homology in their DNA binding domain with vitamin D_3, oestrogen and thyroid hormone receptors. The RARs are characterised by three structural domains consisting of a highly conserved DNA binding domain [C], a less conserved C-terminal ligand-binding domain [E], and a poorly conserved N-terminal region [A/B] which is involved in activation or repression of target gene expression (Fig. 10.6(b)). This work was pioneered by two groups who independently reported the cloning of the RARs (Evans, 1988; Green and Chambon, 1988; reviewed by De Luca, 1991). Retinoids are known to alter gene expression by their interaction with the E region of a given RAR protein. The RAR retinoid complex binds via the DNA binding domain C which contains cysteine-rich 'zinc fingers', to cognate DNA sequences called retinoic acid response elements (RAREs) situated near the promoter region of the target gene. While it may not be surprising that the respective ligands for this receptor 'superfamily' have pronounced effects on cellular differentiation and proliferation, it should be realised that retinoic acid has no affinity for the ligand binding domains of the other members of the family. Some of the genes activated by RARs could also be activated by other members of the family, via recognition by appropriate but again different responsive DNA elements. Six human RAR subtypes have been identified to date. These are designated RAR $\alpha\beta\gamma$ and RXR $\alpha\beta\gamma$. Each subtype exists in several isoforms which arise from alternate splicing and are designated by subscripts, for example RARγ_1. Due to considerable research using molecular biology and immunohistochemistry, the pattern of expression of subtypes and isoforms has been described in detail in numerous embryonic and adult tissues. In addition to their presence, much is also known about the regulation of these proteins and their ability to form heterodimers with auxiliary proteins.

Besides these *cis*-acting nuclear transactivating factors, retinoic acid also binds with high but different affinities to two cytosolic retinoic acid binding proteins, CRABP I and CRABP II, which belong to a family of small serum and cytoplasmic binding proteins associated with the transport and metabolism of low-molecular-weight lipophilic substances. The CRABPs have a molecular weight of 15 kDa and have been cloned from human skin. Retinoic acid causes a

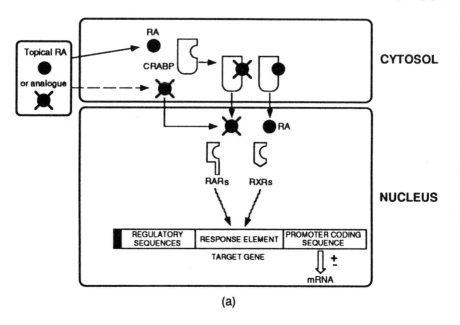

(a)

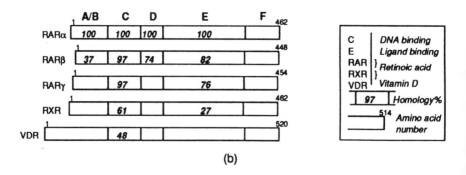

(b)

Fig. 10.6. Retinoid activity: binding to retinoic acid receptors

marked induction of CRABP II mRNA in human skin fibroblasts *in vitro*. The role of these proteins is unclear, but they may act as a shuttle giving the cell access to graded levels of retinoic acid. The over-expression of CRABP II in psoriasis (Didierjean *et al.*, 1991) has been considered as a cause of the hyperproliferative state of the keratinocyte, which essentially finds itself in an environment deficient in retinoids. Independently of a pathological role for CRABP II, retinoids which do not bind to the CRABPs still possess potent biological activities (Darmon *et al.*, 1989). In order to define the roles of these binding proteins further, selective ligands for the six RAR and RXR subtypes would be useful. Despite the relatively high sequence homology in the ligand-binding domains of the RARs, selective ligands have been described. A cursory appraisal of the chemical structures of these ligands and their comparison with compounds such as retinoic acid or CD 367, which have no selectivity, allows the following observations to be made:

(a) Full aromatisation of the linker unit into a naphthalene unit imparts $\alpha \beta$ selectivity.
(b) Introduction of polar units into the linker unit confers α selectivity.
(c) Increased degree of polarity in the lipophilic domain results in γ selectivity.

The structure–binding relationships just described are based on receptor–ligand interactions *in vitro* using competition binding assays. These data are obtained using nucleosol fractions from cells transfected with the respective RAR cDNAs contained in an appropriate expression vector. If, however, these same selective ligands are studied in a transactivation assay, the selectivity ratios can change. A transactivation assay involves co-transfection of gene constructs for both the RAR under study and a reporter gene which contains a cognate DNA response element for the RAR driving a chloramphenicol acetyltransferase (CAT) gene. This type of assay explores a given ligand's ability to bind to and to activate transcription by the protein under study (see Table 10.6). As these studies are carried out in intact cultured cells, endogenous RARs can interfere with the assay. It has been reported that $RAR\gamma_1$ can inhibit transcription modulated by ligand-activated $RAR\alpha$. Complex interactions between these receptor proteins, including autoregulation, may serve to control precisely the activity of retinoic acid in a spatio-temporal manner. This would better explain the idea that a gradient of retinoic acid controls embryonic development (Eichele and Thaller, 1987), since a concentration gradient of retinoic acid, made available to the cell through either local metabolic production or the presence of requisite binding proteins, is probably too crude to explain the precision of retinoic acid action in the control of morphogenesis (see Fig. 10.1).

The interaction between the transactivating proteins may serve to regulate more precisely the actions of retinoic acid and retinoids in general. A most interesting observation concerns the RXR family. The shape of its natural ligand, 9-*cis*-retinoic acid, is different from that of the ligands which only bind

Table 10.6. RAR α, β, γ binding constants and transcription potentials for selective RAR agonists

Compound	K_i (nM)[a]			AC_{50} (nM)[b]		
	α	β	γ	α	β	γ
Retinoic acid	15	4	3	2.1	3.6	2.5
Am 580	8	131	450	0.36	25	28
CD 2019[c]	920	26	160	20	4	47
CD 437[c]	>6000	>2000	77	140	28	7
CD 367	5.3	3	1.3	0.23	0.37	0.25

[a]Calculated in nM from IC_{50} values obtained in competition binding assay. The receptors were isolated from COS 7 cells transfected with RARα, RARβ or RARγ expression vectors.
[b]Concentration giving half-maximal transactivation using HeLa cells transfected with RAR and CAT reporter gene constructs.
[c]See Fig. 10.5. Adapalene: CD 2019; adamantyl replaced by methyl cyclohexyl, CD 437; methoxy replaced by phenol.

with high affinity to the RARs. This may be understood by comparison of the low sequence homology of the ligand-binding domains of these proteins. Some insight into the significance of these interactions can be obtained by studying the pharmacological properties of the selective agonists. The substances listed in Table 10.6 are considered to be such compounds.

DITHRANOL (ANTHRALIN)

Clinical indication: Stable plaque psoriasis.

Local side-effects: Irritation and coloration of non-lesional skin and nails; staining of cloth.

Since the turn of the century this dihydroxy-anthracene derivative has been widely used for the topical treatment of psoriasis. An extensive literature describes its use alone or in combination with corticosteroids, and tar, with or without UV light. Several reviews cover the subject adequately (Kemény et al., 1990; Shroot, 1991) and the purpose of this section is to acquaint the reader with aspects of the pharmacology which give rise to a new rationale for drug design and therapy.

Figure 10.7 illustrates the chemical structure of anthralin and its decomposition products. Being an anthrone, anthralin has an inherent chemical instability mainly towards oxygen and light. In view of these properties, it is not surprising that the inconvenient effects of anthralin are staining of skin and clothes, which result from the oxidation at carbon-10, producing stable, highly coloured free radicals. On the other hand, the biological activity of the drug is related to this same chemical property in that biological oxidation of anthralin is very rapid and the drug is thought to act via inhibition of mitochondrial respiration. Until recently, anthralin was considered to be essentially an

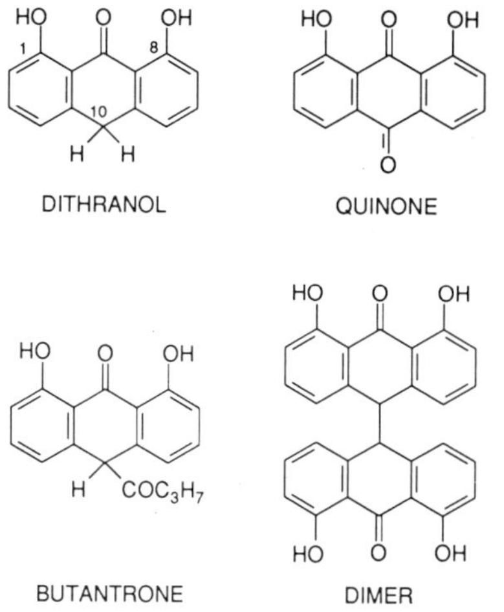

Fig. 10.7.

antiproliferative agent, modulating DNA synthesis via the inhibition of keratinocyte respiration. We cannot exclude the possibility that these effects, as well as many others reported for anthralin such as altered expression of keratins, eicosanoids, histamine and calmodulin (Kemény et al., 1990), may be consequences of a more specific action. An attractive idea relates to a key role for epidermal growth factor (EGF) receptors in the action. In normal human keratinocytes in culture, anthralin was found to decrease the binding of labelled EGF to its receptor and also to inhibit the expression of keratinocyte TGFα mRNA. This finding may lead to studies of the influence of anthralin on the growth factor and cytokine pathways that may regulate epidermal hyperplasia. However, the cell respiratory pathway is by far the most sensitive to dithranol.

Most of the chemical modifications carried out on the anthralin molecule result in products which are less irritating but also less active. Most changes left the reactivity at carbon-10 intact, as the early extensive work of Krebs and Schaltinger postulated that the minimal structure for activity comprised a methylene group at this position and free phenolic functions on carbon-1 and carbon-8. The clinical success of butantrone demonstrates that these requirements are not mandatory. As we saw earlier, the question posed for the medicinal chemist and pharmacologist seeking to improve the therapeutic index in this series is whether efficacy and side-effects can be separated. Clinically, a positive answer has been given by the introduction in the 1980s of short contact therapy and more convenient cream formulations. This scheme, proposed by Schaefer, involves limiting the time that skin is exposed to the drug, the excess being washed out after a treatment lasting 10–60 minutes as opposed to standard overnight (12 hours) application before taking a bath.

Studies of skin permeation showed that short contact was sufficient to permit the drug to penetrate the barrier composed of metabolically hyperactive psoriatic plaques. In that same time, clinically unaffected skin was exposed to less drug and in consequence fewer side-effects were seen (Schaefer, 1985). The clinical advantages of short contact therapy may also apply with new derivatives such as butantrone, which may be a pro-drug of dithranol. Perhaps agents affecting specific growth factors will bring significant advances.

CONCLUSION

Throughout this chapter it has been obvious that the drugs in the armoury of the dermatologist are generally very effective but may have severe side-effects. It still remains for the drug hunters to find safe medication for the treatment of diseases that have long affected mankind. Hampered by a lack of relevant animal models and a plethora of culture models, molecular skin pharmacology is a late-comer. The next 10 years should see the reaping of benefits accrued from studies with transgenic animals expressing aspects of skin diseases which are today only found in man. The identification and characterisation of high-affinity specific receptor targets in the skin will also help drug designers to use molecular modelling more effectively. Finally, to reiterate the opening remarks in this chapter, the above approach for the chemist and pharmacologist will not be relevant without sound clinical pharmacology, which will continue to be the centre of gravity for discovery in dermatology for the foreseeable future.

REFERENCES

Bodor N (1984) Soft drugs: principles and methods for the design of safe drugs. *Medical Research Review* **4**, 449–469.
Darmon M, Rocher M, Cavey MT, Martin B, Rabilloud T, Delescluse C, Bailly J, Eustache J, Jamoulle JC, Nedoncelle P and Shroot B (1989) Affinity of retinoids for nuclear receptors correlates with biological activity by absence of correlation with CRABP binding. In: Reichert U and Shroot B (eds) *Pharmacology of Retinoids in the Skin*, Vol. 3, pp. 56–64. Basel: Karger.
De Luca LM (1991) Retinoids and their receptors in differentiation, embryogenesis and neoplasia. *FASEB Journal* **5**, 2924–2933.
Didierjean L, Durand B and Saurat JH (1991) Cellular retinoic acid-binding protein type 2 mRNA is overexpressed in human psoriatic skin as shown by in situ hybridization. *Biochemical and Biophysical Research Communications* **180**, 204–208.
Eichele G and Thaller C (1987) Characterization of concentration gradients of a morphogenetically active retinoid in the chick limb bud. *Journal of Cell Biology* **105**, 1917–1923.

Elias P (1983) Epidermal lipids, barrier function, and desquamation. *Journal of Investigative Dermatoloty* (Suppl.) **80**, 44–49.

Evans RM (1988) The steroid and thyroid hormone receptor superfamily. *Science* **240**, 889–895.

Green S and Chambon P (1988) Nuclear receptors enhance our understanding of transcription regulation. *Trends in Genetics* **4**, 309–314.

Kemény L, Ruzicka T and Braun-Falco O (1990) Dithranol: a review of the mechanism of action in the treatment of psoriasis vulgaris. *Skin Pharmacology* **3**, 1–20.

Klaus M, Bollag W, Hyber P and Kung W (1983) Sulfur-containing arotinoids, a new class of retinoids. *European Journal of Medical Chemistry* **18**, 425–429.

Kligman AM, Grove GL, Hirose R and Leyden JJ (1986) Topical tretinoin for photoaged skin. *Journal of the American Academy of Dermatology* **15**, 836–859.

Maibach HI, Feldmann RJ, Milby T and Serat W (1971) Regional variation in percutaneous penetration in man. *Archives of Environmental Health* **23**, 208–211.

Schaefer H (1985) Short-contact therapy. *Archives of Dermatology* **121**, 1505–1512.

Shroot B (1989) A strategy for discovery of new retinoid-like substances. In: Reichert U and Shroot B (eds) *Pharmacology of Retinoids in the Skin*, Vol. 3, pp. 270–277. Basel: Karger.

Shroot B (1991) Anthralin. In: Roenigk HH Jr and Maibach HI (eds) *Psoriasis*, 2nd edn, pp. 481–499. New York: Dekker.

Stoughton RB (1992) Vasoconstrictor assay: specific applications. In: Maibach HI and Surber C (eds) *Topical Corticosteroids*, pp. 42–53. Basel: Karger.

Straumfjord JV (1943) Vitamin A. Its effect in acne. *Northwestern Medicine* **42**, 219–225.

Stüttgen G (1986) Historical perspectives of tretinoin. *Journal of the American Academy of Dermatology* **15**, 735–739.

Wertz PW, Madison KC and Downing DT (1989) Covalently bound lipids of human stratum corneum. *Journal of Investigative Dermatology* **92**, 109–111.

Williams K (1985) Importance of drug enantiomers in clinical pharmacology. *Drugs* **4**, 333–354.

SUGGESTED FURTHER READING

Greaves MW and Shuster S (eds) (1989a) *Pharmacology of the Skin I. Pharmacology of Skin Systems, Autocoids in Normal and Inflamed Skin*. Berlin: Springer-Verlag.

Greaves MW and Shuster S (eds) (1989b) *Pharmacology of the Skin II. Methods, Absorption, Metabolism and Toxicity, Drugs and Diseases*. Berlin: Springer-Verlag.

Index

tumour necrosis factor α (TNFα), 65,
   132, 137
  accumulation rate, 143
  in epidermis, 137–8
  immune response effects, 137
tumour necrosis factor β (TNFβ), 138
tumours
  growth of solid, 103
  invasion, 103–5
  TNFα actions, 137
tyrosinase, 57, 60–1
  activity in black skin, 61
  control points in regulation, 61
  genes, 60
  post-translational glycosylation, 61
  mRNA splicing, 61
  testosterone effects, 67
  UVR stimulation, 64
tyrosinase gene
  tanning response, 64
  transcription, 61
tyrosinase synthesis
  and tanning ability, 65
  UVA therapy, 64
tyrosinase-related protein 1 (TRP-1), 60,
   62
tyrosinase-related protein 2 (TRP-2), 62
tyrosinase-related protein (TRP genes),
   61–2
tyrosine kinase, 68

ultra-high sulphur keratins, 48
ultraviolet radiation (UVR)
  absorption, 7
  cell damage, 6–7
  delayed action response, 63–4
  effects, 63–5
  glycosaminoglycan effects, 106

mutagen, 181
  protection against, 55
utricles, 201–2

vectors, 173
versican, 90, 93, 94, 97
vimentin, 27
  gene location on chromosome, 32
  genes, 32
  homopolymeric filaments, 28
vitamin A, 176
  acne treatment, 199
vitamin D₃, 55, 63
  production by keratinocytes, 65
vitiligo, 6, 71
  familial, 15

Waardenburg's syndrome, 183–4
warts, viral, 14
wax esters, 152, 154
  sebum content, 155
waxy coats, 151
whiteheads, 156
wool
  keratins, 25
  microfibrillar keratins, 35–6
  structure, 2
wound healing, 5, 75, 100–2
  clot formation, 100
  factors for ending phase, 102
  osteonectin, 107
  TNFα actions, 137
  tumour growth, 103

yeast artificial chromosomes (YAC), 42

zinc deficiency, 16
zymogens, 124

Index compiled by Jill C. Halliday